TABLE OF CONTENTS

Foreward 2

Chapter 1 – The Beginning 4

Chapter 2 – Living with a bad back 32

Chapter 3 – My worst Hospital experience ever 42

Chapter 4 – October 2012 51

Chapter 5 – November 2012 63

Chapter 6 – December 2012 72

Chapter 7 – January 2013 75

Chapter 8 – March 2013 90

Chapter 9 – July 2013 100

Chapter 10 – The last FIVE Months of 2013 110

Chapter 11 – The RInging in of the new year 123

Chapter 12 – Sunday 26th January 2014............................... 137

Chapter 13 – Guilt and the low esteem................................ 144

Resources 159

FOREWARD

I suffer from an immune disease called Polymyalgia Rheumatica. Yes it is a bloody mouthful to say but those of us who suffer with this disease call it PMR. Normally this disease affects people in their 70's. When you are diagnosed with it at the age of 55, when your golden years are supposed to be before you… it really can have a huge affect on not just your physical well-being but also your mental health.

At times I don't know what I would have done, if it had not been for my family… they have supported, helped and been with me, every step of the way. Without their support, their love, I don't know how I would have got through some of those days… especially the days when I could hardly move and the aches and pains didn't subside, no matter how many pain killers I took.

Thank you, I know this illness can't be easy on you all, but thanks for sticking around and not abandoning me... and I love you all so much

CHAPTER 1 – THE BEGINNING

My story starts way back in 1988, when I thought I was actually Wonder Woman without those ghastly – hold-it-in-at-all-costs – star studded knickers and that fake gold crown that looks like it was the prototype of a Christmas cracker hat; and I thought I had her strength to help move a washing machine... Oh yes those were the days, when I had to prove women are equal to men and we are not some blonde bimbos incapable of lifting a drawing pin. Yes the days of chaining ourselves to fences were well and truly over and we now had real rights.

Well me and Dishface (the ex, who we won't even talk about, because if I let rip into him, then I would either be sued, have an injunction imposed on me, and raise my blood pressure to dangerous levels) lifted this a new washing machine through the front door... just as we were about to turn to manoeuvre the tight bend to the kitchen... snap, bang, scream… my back went.

Having a 4-year-old who was constantly on the go... a bad back was something I could well do without. It was hard enough running around the house at times trying to catch the little blighter who could run faster than me and chuckled so hard that you couldn't stop laughing at him, let alone trying to run, whilst looking as if you had just had an accident in your knickers and doing you best 'I'm as pissed as a parrot John Wayne look.'

Painkillers... where are they? Give them to me quick? Stupidly I thought a couple of Paracetamol would do the trick... along with a couple of Ibuprofen to kill this pain, but no my old back was having none of it... By the time the morning came, after not being able to sleep properly and popping painkillers like Smarties, I was still doubled up in pain and was taken to the doctors who then told me to go straight to the hospital. I was examined by a couple of the A & E doctors, who then called for the some specialist and that was it; I was admitted into hospital and put in traction... Yes nearly 4 whole days of laying flat on your back... staring at a white ceiling, is enough for you to go insane.

But the hardest part, for me, was not being in pain but when my little soldier came to see me and I had to say goodbye. It broke my heart. Mind you on his first visit, he did think it was great fun to swing on the weights that were hanging over the edge of the bed. When I screamed out in agony he soon got off. My God that child was beginning to remind me of Tarzan by the minute.

Day four arrived in that hospital and the Doctor arrived in the afternoon to examine me and said that the nurses were going to remove me from traction and that if I could walk unassisted by the next day... I could go home... YIPPEE!

That was it... no way was I going to be in that hospital another day than I needed to be. I now became a woman on a mission – 'Operation Get Home' was now in full implementation and needed to be finalized by the end of the following afternoon. James Bond move over. Jane Bond 007½, now had the licence to kill should anybody get her way and stop her going home.

There I was in agony forcing a smile and getting about unassisted, whilst profoundly swearing in the toilets and crumpling on the toilet seat counting down those minutes and seconds until I heard that Doctor say 'Go Home'.... and I was doing all of this whilst making sure that no-one was in those other cubicles to report me. I was going home and that was it... pain, agony, or whatever else was thrown at me I would take in my stride, nothing was going to force me to stay in that hospital one second longer than I needed to. That is one thing you do learn by having a baby... the art of breathing to take the edge off those sharp stabbing pains, and those ante-natal lesions were now worth their weight in gold whilst dealing with the pain of sciatica and a slipped disc.

That very afternoon, the Doctor was pleased with my progress. In fact I think he was rather amazed at how well I got about without grimacing too much... little did he know about my heavy breathing and swearing antics in the toilets, because I'm sure if he did he would've made me stay a little longer.

Oh I couldn't pull the wool over my Dad's eyes though as he came to collect me. He knew exactly what I did to get out of there because when I got in the car after being discharged I said, 'It doesn't hurt as much as it did when I came in here, but at least I can move a bit now. Get me out of here and get me home.'

To help me out my parents allowed us to move in there until I felt better, but that only lasted a couple of weeks, because Dishface decided to play up, yet again. It was getting to be a regular thing with him now and my Dad thought it might be better all-round if I went home and he and my mum came over to help me in the day, when he was not in the vicinity. I think my dad was at breaking point with him and didn't want me to be in the midst of a row, because my dad couldn't and wouldn't hold his tongue much longer.

Eventually time passed and I was back to full health... yes I would get a little niggle of pain now and again in my back but nothing that warranted me to take to my bed. Life was good in the health department; it sucked however in the all other departments... Just a couple of months after I was released from hospital my father died suddenly. One minute he was out shopping with us, next he had a major stroke. Before being transferred to the ambulance, he had another turn and died on the floor and was revived with CPR. I arrived just as he was being revived and once the paramedics got him stable, he was transferred to the ambulance and my mum and I were racing through the streets of Medway, with my father now in a critical condition, heading for our local hospital. He never regained consciousness and stayed in a coma for just over a week before suffering another stroke which was too much for his body to endure and he passed away peacefully.

The care that the hospital gave my father was exemplary; he was kept comfortable, washed morning and night and monitored at regular intervals. You could not criticise the level of care. The compassion and empathy, show to us his family, was beyond the level of care expected. Whether they knew it was just a matter of time or not, I don't know, but they made time for us. They even fed us at times and answered all questions in a manner so that we could understand what was happening.

During this time, our hopes were raised for a couple of days, when there was slight improvement in his condition. He was still in a coma but the doctors were talking about transferring him to Woolwich hospital who were experts in strokes, but those hopes were sadly dashed.

Helping mum arrange a funeral was something I had to do… he was my dad and I had to do right by him. And I tried to suppress the grief as much as I could, but I was finding times hard. I couldn't talk to my mum, she was suffering, so I bottled everything up… until there was time for me to deal with my own emotions. I just went through the next few months totally oblivious as to what was really going in this big wide world. Dishface was as much help as a fart in a thunderstorm to put it bluntly.

Now if that wasn't enough to make any person want to throw the towel in.... my relationship with Dishface finally came to an end. I could take no more and decided kick him and his backside out of the door.

The years of 1988 and 1989 were not good years for me, firstly with back problems and then having to deal with the trials and tribulations of a divorce whilst grieving for a father that I loved dearly. Apart from still suffering from twinges of back pain, I also had the emotional side of a breakup to deal with; whilst trying to play mum and dad to a little boy who was just about to turn 5. Times were not easy that's for sure but I knew I either had to be a single-parent living hand to mouth, because the words 'child maintenance' sent Dishface in a real old lather so much so that the threat of court action, would mean him being out of work once again and making a fortnightly visit to the DHSS to sign on, until the threat had passed.

There was only my mum left to help me, and as she had just lost her husband and soul-mate, I couldn't put my worries on her too heavily, as she was also grieving for my dad, even though she never complained and would volunteer at every given chance to babysit. But living on part-time money, with no maintenance was getting harder by the minute... so the only option was full-time work.

I hated the thought of leaving my son every day... the prospect of not being the one to walk him to school and to be there the moment he came out of school, felt like a dagger permanently stabbing my heart, without any let-up. But needs must, as they say. To make it easier on both myself and my mum, I moved back home with her. Luckily the move didn't cause too much havoc with regards to my son's education, as he had only just started full-time school... so all-in-all the move back home turned out to be quite a smooth transition, not just for him but for me as well.

Within a couple of weeks of being back at home, with my mum and son, I applied for a job with our local Police Constabulary. I was overjoyed to get an interview... I had been out of the office environment with regards to work for nearly seven years and even though the interview went well, I didn't want to get my hopes up and then feel all disappointed when I got the rejection letter, which I was convinced I was going to get.

But, that interview must have gone better than I had thought, because within days of I was offered the position and the starting salary was far better than I expected. Initially the job offer was by phone with written confirmation being sent in the post. Finally my life and that of my son was turning into something that had a brighter future ahead of it, than it had just a few weeks previously.

I moved on with my life... mum was great and would babysit for me so that I could go out with friends and meet new people. Then, after vowing never to become involved in a full-on relationship, I found myself a lovely man to whom I am now married to and life couldn't be any sweeter.

Weeks passed and this fantastic guy was still in my life, the months went by and then we decided to live together... Things just got better and better and we were one happy little family.

Then in 1993, whilst playing around chasing my son, I stumbled and tore all the tendons and ligaments in my ankle. I couldn't walk on it and after a few weeks I had to have ultrasound treatment on it... as well as having it strapped up, because my ankle was starting to turn inwards and they wanted to stretch those tendons a little to make them more pliable. This went on for months and months... with the problem escalating, due to the fact that my back was now beginning to suffer and started to hurt like crazy again.

I was now living with a man I loved dearly; I was working in a job I loved, which I knew had great opportunities for me to progress further with promotions within the department I was working in or other departments. I was fed up and I wanted to get back to work. Surely there must be a light at the end of this tunnel, mustn't there and the day will come soon when I can walk again into work with no problems? Surely things couldn't get any worse, could they?

Watch out incoming, as they say... yes the bombshell of all bombshells –talk about Weapons of Mass Destruction, this was the bomb that would annihilate everything in its path – this one was the killer of all hope,...yes through the post came a letter saying that due to my sickness time, which was now reaching close to 5 months, I had to go to see the Force Doctor and could I ring to make an appointment and the letter went on to explain that my employment status as to whether I would still be employed or not rested on his medical assessment.

I couldn't drive at all during that period, which was again bloody annoying: housebound, walking on crutches with my car sitting outside gathering dust. So the appointment was made at a time when it was convenient for my partner to take me, as he was a shift-worker. I picked up the phone and made the appointment, for a couple of weeks later hoping by then my ankle would start to improve now that is strapped up tightly. As for the bad back, I would have doped myself up on painkillers and acted OK, remember I am now super-trained in grimacing whilst smiling... but nothing I did with regards to my ankle made it strong enough for me to be able walk without the aid of crutches yet alone put my full weight on it, and so off to Force Headquarters I headed for my examination with the Force Doctor hoping that the worst possible outcome from that examination didn't materialise, and I lost my job.

It wasn't long after the appointment that his medical assessment report was sent to the Head of my department, along with a copy sent to me at my home address, and it stated that upon examination he could not see me returning to work in the near future as my ankle injury had triggered off an old injury that was now causing me as much agony as my ankle and recommended that I should be medically retired... Retired at 35... Surely not?

Over the following years, I learnt what I could and couldn't do? I encountered more sleepless nights than a mother with a new born baby at times. One minute I could sleep then the next I would wake up in complete agony. Time taught me to do what I could do and to how to spot the warning signs... those first twinges of pain, which shone like big red flashing traffic lights... and I knew when those pains appeared, STOP WHAT YOU ARE DOING AND TAKE IT EASY.

When my back decided it was not going to play ball, if I managed to get a few hours solid sleep at night it was a bonus... but things could have been worse. There are a lot of other people who are in a worse situation than I am. Don't grumble... just take the medication, do what you can do and take what ill-health throws at you, on the chin.

Then in 1996, crash bang wallop. I was walking up the garden path and sneezed. Just me doing one simple little 'atishoo', like I did many times before without any problems, was now the onset of another back problem. Who would have believed that you could slip another disc, by sneezing? Never in a million years did I think that would happen... and after nearly 3 weeks of terrible pain and sciatica I was taken back into hospital with the prospect of having to have surgery.

Travelling in that ambulance wasn't bad... gas and air... I never had gas and air when I gave birth to my son, so have never experienced it the pleasures of it... but that trip to the hospital that day was like travelling on a cloud... being whisked away and feeling all sleepy, giddy and happy and not giving a shite about what was happening to me... Plus it got rid of the sharp stabbing pains... I was in heaven after 3 weeks of pure agony.

The examinations, the scans, the X-rays, laying in the accident and emergency department waiting for a bed, seemed never ending. I was admitted to A & E in the afternoon and didn't get to the ward until very late that night. Yes the usual prods and pokes and questions... FFS I have been through this in A & E why do I have to repeat myself? You have injected me with stuff to take away the pain, you have given me tablets to ease the pain... now I want to sleep, something I haven't quite managed to do in the last 3 weeks other than catnaps, so I wished these people who are trying to get me better would leave me alone to sleep. All these thoughts were running through my mind but I just didn't have the energy to moan or complain or say anything for that matter, I just wanted to sleep. Night came and the new day dawned and I was in a lot less pain than I had been evening before but I was still so tired. I could have slept for England. The thought of having to get out of that bed, is something I didn't relish at all. But I had to and I was parched, craving for a coffee, but the nurse informed me that the doctor was doing his rounds and wanted to see how I was and discuss what was going to happen next. No offer of coffee and she had taken the bloody water jug as well. Then they arrived, just like buses, you wait ages and then three turn up at once, and so the medical examination began and a group of student doctors were then ushered in to watch this medical examination.

Being told by a dishy Doctor, that very morning, who himself suffered from a severe case of bloody cold hands, that the operating room awaits me, is definitely not my idea of fun, or playing doctors and nurses for that matter. 'My dear,' he said, 'I think this is the only alternative at the moment for you. You see the disc you have just slipped has not protruded to the left or the right, like your other disc, but it has gone central and is pressing on your sciatic nerve which is causing you this severe pain and the numbness in your right leg.'

As I lay there, on the most uncomfortable bed ever, shot full of painkillers and high as a kite, the Doctor started to manipulate my leg and the pain started to subside, whether it was the pain killers kicking in I don't know but I was gradually being able to move better. Perhaps it was the fear of the scalpel that made me feel better. I don't know but the object of my goal was to go home.

Help what do I do, talk about I'm a celebrity get me out of here... I was pleading with my husband to take me home. Frantic... you don't know the half of it. I was laying there like a Chivers jelly wobbling all over the place. I was so frightened that my knees were actually playing a tune, where they were knocking together and I had a husband that said it is best if the operation is carried out now. Great you wait until I am home and you will be in for the high jump... Visions of me making him chocolate mousse, with ex-lax and leaving the bathroom 'toilet roll free' were running through my mind. Remember guys, don't upset a woman when she is in pain and having a bout of PMT. Because you will come off the worse, believe me.

Now it dawned on me why my request to the nurse for a cup of coffee fell on stony ground, it was because I was going to be sliced and diced.

So apart from laying there gagging for a drink, I was now facing the prospect of spending the following six weeks either standing or laying and not being allowed to sit, as well as having a panic attack about being operated on. When it comes to operations and painful procedures, and believe me I only visit the dentist when I can't stand the pain no longer, I am the world's biggest coward. And here I was now facing my worst nightmare ever... being operated on. I had previously had one operation on my hand to remove a ganglion but that was sprung on me so quick, that I don't think I had the chance to panic and it meant only staying in hospital for a few hours after surgery....but this... No I didn't want this operation, but unfortunately I felt pressured. Not just by the hospital but by my other half who thought at that precise time it was for the best.

I don't like to hear about tragic accidents, but another person's accident saved me that day. You see, out there in this wild world someone decided to drive somewhere and they were tragically involved in an accident which now meant that the hospital was in urgent need of the operating theatre to treat people who were involved in this accident and therefore my back operation was to be put on hold as there was improvement in my condition, and my operation would have to be rebooked. Brilliant... no knock-out drops today then.

Then came the best news ever... The kind Doctor believed that, as my manoeuvrability was better than the day before when I was admitted, I could go home and rest.... I don't think that was the entire reason for them letting me go home, I had heard the nurses mention the bed shortages they had and how they had patients waiting in A & E for admittance to that particular ward. I don't care what the real reasons were; it still meant I was going home.

That was it ... like a bullet out of a gun I was out of there.

Of course when I was admitted all I had for attire was my nightie, old dressing gown and threadbare slippers. These were the first things he grabbed to get some clothes on me because it was when I trying to get out of the bath that my back finally decided to give up the ghost and an ambulance needed to be called. That morning when he arrived, all he bought with him was the post…men.

Of course when the news came that I was finally coming home, he knew I wouldn't agree to him going home and getting me some clothes, just in case they changed their minds. There I was, still in my nightwear, gingerly walking the corridors of the hospital to the car park at a snail's pace. When he decided to leave me at the entrance of A & E and drive the car up to there and get me in and take me home. Mind you I was thankful that with the post he bought a packet of cigarettes and a lighter… because believe me by that time I was prepared to commit mass murder for a ciggie. There I was parked on a bench outside A & E, in my old slippers, which the toe had gone through, my old toweling dressing gown that had practically every thread pulled and a nightie that had holes under the armpits, when this young copper asks walks up to me and says, 'Are you ok ma'am. Should you be out here in this cold weather?' I thought this is it, if he starts to grab my arm and march me back in that hospital I will be done for assaulting a copper... because there was no way I was going back in there now they'd let me go. By luck hubby pulled up in the car and I was finally on my way home.

Hubby knew there and then, once they let me escape there was no way in this world that I would agree to go back and be operated on. I went back for the outpatients appointments, but eventually when they realised that I was not going to consent to an operation, they were happy to discharge me completely and told me to return should ever I lose control of my bowels or bladder as this could be a sign that there is more pressure on the nerves in my back. Luckily, to this day that has never happened. Thank God. Their decision to discharge me and my decision not to have the operation was a good thing, because I was told a couple of years down the line, by a locum doctor, that the operation would have been 50/50. And out of that 50 percent chance it failed there was a 20 percent chance I could end up in a worse state.

I was home and even though my back ached at times and my sciatic nerve gives me gyp... upon hearing what that Locum said, I was so thankful that I had never agreed to have that operation... If the odds had been 80 percent chance I would be better and 20 per cent chance that I would stay the same... those odds I could have dealt with... but not the ones they were offering. The fear of being paralysed or having to spend the rest of my life in a wheelchair is something that I didn't want to even think about let alone contemplate.

In 2000, through my husband's employers private medical insurance, I was admitted to Fawkham Manor Hospital as a private patient with my own room with en-suite and a menu that had wine on it... Fancy getting told off in a private hospital... I was... simply because I didn't ask for pain relief. The nurse said, 'This hospital is not the NHS you know, you don't have to suffer here. If you are in pain, press the buzzer and we will give you some pain relief.' That was it, no suffering for me... I was only in there for 2 nights but my god did that hospital care for their patients in such a courteous and qualified manner and they knew exactly how to look after their patients. That kind of treatment made the patients feel at ease and not so fearful of what was going to happen. There was no rushing between patients... there were nurses allocated to a set number of patients and when they came on and came off of duty they would pop their head around the door and say, 'Good Morning' or 'Good Night' as well as enquiring how you felt. There was no rush to end the conversation... they took their time and listened. If only the NHS could be like this.

As years rolled by, I knew my capabilities... what I could and couldn't do with regards to my back and sciatica... moving washing machines was definitely off of the list. And I knew what to do the moment those niggling twinges of pain come back... rest, painkillers and pray like crazy that the pain goes away soon. Sleeping was still a problem and still is today... and when you can't sleep for more than a few hours, the next day you are walking around, like a zonked out zombie. Luckily, sleeping during the next day was one option I could and still to this day, take.

When the nights are full of pain, they seem so long. It seems as if the whole world had been in slumber for years... not just minutes. And seriously do you know what really gets you? When you are so dog-tired and you see others sleeping like a baby, and you know full well you can't because to lie there just puts your body in pain.

One of the ways I have found to relieve my bad back is to soak in a hot bath... let the hot water melt away those pains and make those muscles that are so tense, where they are so constricted, caused by me holding myself in such a way that it caused practically every muscle to tense up.

However, help at times is needed, to get in and out of the bath. But on one particular hot-bath-soak occasion, not long after I was released from hospital the second time, my dearly beloved decided to help me get in the bath and then shoot off to Tesco's. Now how the hell was I supposed to get out? And what made matters even more intolerable is that I didn't know he had any plans to go to Tesco's; let alone go. I couldn't believe the situation I was in; there I was calling him at the top of my voice and getting no reply. The only solution it seemed, was to stay in the bath, become a prune and wait until he heard my cries. That particular episode taught me how to turn on the hot tap to get more hot water in the bath as the temperature of the bath water was plummeting. But after being wrinkled like a 100-year-old person, I eventually managed to get the assistance so desperately needed to get out of that friggin bath.

Roll on 2012, still managing to evade any form of surgery or re-admittance to my local hospital, when damn, drat and blast there I was trying to kneel on floor and all of a sudden I got a very severe sharp pain in my right knee and my knee gave out. Ouch... the pain was so intense and had no intention of subsiding so the only alternative left open to me was to call my GP for an appointment.

Off to the doctors the following day, stinking of Deep Heat and hobbling. Upon examination of my knee I was told I needed an X-ray done as she could feel the inflammation and thought I could have Osteoarthritis in the knee. So armed with an X-ray form and blood tests forms in my hand, home I went.

Getting to Medway Hospital, via bus is a flaming nightmare, you have to go into Chatham change buses and when you are hobbling and it hurts like crazy to put weight on your knee, getting on and off buses doesn't help.

Anyway hubby had an appointment with our GP early October, and decided to take the day off... any excuse. He said he would take me to hospital early in the morning, I found out that the X-ray department opened at 8.30 am and the blood test place at 7 am so we arrived early and got seen very promptly. That was it, visit done and dusted in less than an hour, knees were X-rayed and blood tests done...

Oh don't talk about blood tests... unfortunately, I am one of these people who doesn't want to part with their blood, so 9 times out of 10, the poor nurse can't use the crease of my arm by the elbow to get blood, like they would do normally... So I either have the option of having it taken from the lower arm or the upper arm. Of course, that is after I have been stabbed a couple of times and they decide they can't do it from the normal place.

Mind you there is one male Phlebotomist, that I have got to know and who knows me and knows exactly where to take my blood from, usually in the lower arm. When I have these tests now he has told me to tell them where the easiest place is and they will take it from there without me having to turn into a pin cushion.

So blood taken, knees having been X-rayed ,all there was left for me to do now is wait for the results... trying to keep the fear of whether this could be the onset of Bone Cancer out of my mind. God Google is your best friend, when you want to know the number of the local takeaway, but it is your worst nightmare when trying self diagnoses as to what could be wrong with you, every site checked had those fearful words... Bone Cancer. And is that the reason why I am in so much agony, with my muscles, bones and why my body aches all the damn time?

I think you now hear so many times about people you know or you have family and friends who have to face cancer and the radical treatment needed so that they can live a few more years or better still be cured, that your mind automatically thinks of the worst possible thing.

Years ago, it seemed such a rare thing to hear… but now… I don't know it just frightens the shite out of you, when something goes wrong with your body.

Cancer doesn't choose poor people, it chooses rich people and poor people and it doesn't matter how much money you have, if cancer is going to get you … it will. And it has left a fear in people's minds…..

Keep calm… don't say a thing… with one thing after another I am beginning to turn into the half-empty glass sort of gal… and not the glass half full person I used to be.

CHAPTER 2 – LIVING WITH A BAD BACK

When you have two slipped discs, and a trapped nerve that has left you with no feeling in the back of your right leg in the upper thigh/buttock region also parts of your right calf, heel and side of foot including the little toe, you have to learn to adjust.

Your ambitions of being a limbo dancer are over... No more tripping the light fantastic for you. You might manage a smooch now and again but as for swinging from a chandelier... forget it. Your body isn't going to get in those positions ever again, believe me.

Sciatica is painful believe me at the best of times... but when you have spasm attacks of a sharp stabbing pain which starts in your right heel and then spreads violently up your sciatic nerve, and with such intensity that it takes your breath away. Sometimes I am lucky these spasms last just a few minutes... but when I get a bad attack it can last for hours. Many a night I am woken up with these spasms and lie there tensing my foot and holding my breath and praying that was the last one... but then the next spasm comes and then the next... When the spasms eventually stop you lie there thinking apprehensively that they could start up again. The pain can be so severe at times that by the end of the attack you are physically and mentally exhausted. And if you are up and about on your feet when these attacks start your leg gives way and you end up having to grab something quick to hold onto.

Throughout the years a few times, I have had these attacks and they have resulted in trips to the hospital or me inflicting another injury on myself.

1994 was the year we decided to move... and it wasn't long after we moved that I was coming down the steps of our back garden and one of these spasmodic pains started. Unfortunately just as I was about to go down to the next step, a sharp pain went down my right leg... that was it I missed the step, twisted my ankle and landed flat on my face. I just knew that I had torn the ligaments in my ankle.

Here we go again, I thought, another load of bloody agro only this time, the other ankle.

From the moment I was born, I was brought up with dogs in the family, and life to me isn't the same unless there is a dog in the home. To me a dog makes a home complete... plus when you are not well they do have excellent pet therapy qualities. Well, we had two dogs... a Heinz 57, who had more breeds in her than the Kennel Club had registered and a 14st Saint Bernard, who was a gentle giant, clumsy but still a gentle giant. As for the clumsy part they say your dog is an extension of you...and yes I am clumsy and accident prone.

There I lay at the bottom of the steps by the back door and the Saint did what I suppose Saints instinctively do...rescue you.

Yes she tried to get me up, by sniffing and licking my face, but I suppose because I didn't leap to my feet promptly enough for her, she decided that she needed to keep me warm... You lay on concrete for what seemed like hours with a Saint Bernard lying on top of you. Keeping me warm... Jesus wept it was friggin summer... I was not warm... I was about to pass out with heat exhaustion...

After a few commands that were being totally ignored at first, she moved. I don't think it was the commands as much that made her move... I think it was because the sun was belting down on her and she couldn't take the heat. But I was thankful to be finally to be free. I struggled indoors by this time, using an ice-pack to stop the swelling was pointless, as by now my foot was swollen like a balloon. Next point of call for me was... yes, you've guessed the answer – a trip to the hospital. After repeating what happened before with the other ankle... the hospital decided to put my foot in plaster for 10 days, to give time for the tendons and ligaments to heal...

Having spent a few hours at the hospital being plastered up and given instructions on how to use crutches I came home... For the first 48 hours you are not allowed to put any weight on the cast... so things were a bit difficult but I managed.

10 days later I returned to the hospital and had the plaster cast removed. Now that was hilarious, my mate took me, and one thing I can't stand is people touching my feet. There I was on

this table when the chap came along with his power tool to remove the cast. It was just like a little circular saw, but the vibration of it cutting through the plaster made me chuckle as it tickled my foot. I just couldn't control myself. In the end the guy, operating this saw, was chuckling with me. As I left he said to me, 'I have never known someone with such sensitive feet.'

Anyway foot was stiff after the cast was removed but after a few days, I was back to normal. Until the next accident happened and I was back visiting those nice people at A & E.

This time, it didn't involve any limbs, requiring medical assistance… it was my face. If you can image it our hall was small… you opened the front door and took two steps and you were going up the stairs. Just to the side of the stairs was a recessed area where we had the hall mirror and where the radiator was housed. Of course this left the corner of the stairs wall, next to the recess with an exposed edge.

On this day, I came through the door and my right leg gave out and again I fell smack up against the radiator and smashed the left side of my face on the corner of the wall and my forehead on the radiator. Hubby was at work, but luckily the next-door-neighbor was home and I went to them and he took me to the hospital. His partner didn't have a bag of peas, but gave me a bag of frozen chips to stop the swelling. And she rang my husband at work and told him what had happened and that I was now on my way to the hospital.

As I arrived at the hospital, I felt bad and my eye was closing... It just looked as if I had been smacked in the side of the face with a baseball bat. After sitting there a short while, my husband turned up... and looked at me shaking his head, as if to say, 'What the fuck have you done now?'

The doctor emerged and there I was now with two men in my company. The doctor showed me the way to the treatment room and as my husband went to get up and come in with me... the doctor told him to wait there and he would call him if needed. As I sat in the chair, it was now getting to the point where it was getting too painful to speak. The doctor kept asking me how I did it, time and time again. I tried to tell him through the pain that I had fallen, but somehow he didn't seem convinced.

An X-ray was ordered for my face and normally they send you out to walk around to the X-ray department yourself, only this time the nurse took me, bypassing my husband altogether. Still the penny had not dropped. She waited whilst the X-ray was performed and then took me straight back to the treatment room.

My face was killing me, the pain was so immense and I could feel my left eye closing more and more and stiffness coming to my cheek and jaw, and to be honest the last thing on my mind was having a bloody good natter, but no this nurse was not having the silent treatment and kept trying to talk to me about things… like where I live, do I work, etc… But all I wanted to do was get rid of this pain and go home and curl up on the settee.

Finally X-ray done and the nurse and I returned to treatment room…still no sign of my husband…what the heck was going on… where had he gone?

The doctor re-appeared and said there was nothing broken and if I wanted I could go home, but he was prepared to admit me, if that is what I wanted. What I wanted? I want to go home you fucking idiot...I wouldn't have been here in the first place if it hadn't been for the persistence of my next-door-neighbor saying I should go to the hospital. What the heck was this doctor on about and then he started to broach the subject of battered women, whilst the nurse then started to hand me leaflets on head injuries and domestic violence in the home.

The penny finally dropped... they must have thought I was a victim of domestic violence... through my now swollen face I tried to tell them they were barking up the wrong tree and it was an accident... but somehow I don't think they were convinced. I wanted to laugh... but I couldn't, it hurt far too much. Me, a battered wife? Never. Anyway they told me to take pain killers and it might be advisable to eat mushy stuff for a few days and take things easy, and that I could go home if I wanted. By this time my sense of humour had now gone into over-drive and I just wanted to burst out laughing at the thought of the hospital thinking my old man had given me a good old clobbering.

As we got into the car, I told him what they had thought had happened to me; and that me saying I had fallen was an excuse for the injuries, because I was in fear of getting another beating.

We looked at each other and chuckled, and he said to me, 'I thought that doctor gave me a look of contempt and I wondered why I wasn't allowed in and when I asked a nurse she said the Doctor will get back to you soon.'

When I got back home and looked into the mirror, I think it was then that I realised just how much of a battered wife I did look.

Even now when I think back on that day, I still laugh my head off, to think whilst he was building the M2 Bridge, I was falling through the door and smashing my face in... an accident he was about to take the blame for.

Of course there has been the obligatory trip of coming down the stairs only to have a sharp pain that makes my right leg give away, and I finalise those last few steps on my posterior, which then turns black and blue.

I think my hubby has finally realised that I am just one big, not literally, accident waiting to happen. I don't intend to hurt myself but my God if something is going to fall on someone it's always me.

So now when I have these pains I make sure I am nowhere near anything that can hurt me… who knows if they suspect him once more, the next time I hurt myself, he could be arrested, charged and jailed before I had the chance to tell them he's not to blame.

When I was a child I was accident prone, and as an adult I have kept that trait with me… only this time the accidents seem to be causing me more pain than I want or need.

But all in all I have learnt what I can do and what I can't, so I know my limitations and don't push them to the point of where I could end up back in any hospital, being patched up, put in plaster cast, or admitted due to them thinking I am a victim of domestic violence.

CHAPTER 3 – MY WORST HOSPITAL EXPERIENCE EVER

Then it had to happen, I suffered the worst hospital experience of my life in 1998. For weeks, even months I had suffered with violent stomach aches and feeling sick... Again like a chicken I refused to go anywhere. Normally being sick seemed to stop the agony. However one day after throwing up... and believe me I could throw up - enough to get England a gold medal with no problems - my usual method of inducing myself to be sick being that of sticking my fingers down my throat, didn't work. I couldn't stop the pain, and I was doubled up in pain. The pain would subside a little and then it would come back with a vengeance. Well a couple of days went by and I was getting no better and eventually, I had to concede that I was ill and agreed to allowing them to call a doctor. The out-of-hour's doctor was called and upon examination wanted me to go to hospital for further investigation. 'Hang on in there sunshine,' I thought... 'I don't do hospitals unless I have to.' And I politely told him to give me a good pain killer and I will be OK. Well he gave me an injection and told my husband to ring our GP when they opened if I wasn't any better. The injection allowed me to sleep for a while but not that long.

Well that was it, I didn't feel better, in fact if anything things were getting worse to the point that I was now on a projectile vomiting mission, even a sip of water would now miraculously transform into a fountain of vomit which left my hubby no alternative but to call our GP who came out immediately. Upon examination and a swift telling-off for not going somewhere sooner, an ambulance was called for me by my GP and off to hospital I went. Yes it was an emergency admittance and apparently I was suffering from Pancreatitis, which by all accounts can be serious and even fatal as they tell me now and apparently it is one of the complaints that alcoholics get. After being examined, drips put in (and that involved at least 25 attempts because the veins in my hands were suffering due to me now being severely dehydrated; it was eventually a sister who managed to get the cannula into the back of what was being becoming an already bruised hand), oxygen blood tests which were painful as they had to take blood from the area of your pulse being done at least twice, the oxygen mask constantly being replaced over my face as soon as I filled the next cardboard kidney bowl full of vomit and doctors coming in and out as if they had never seen a woman vomit as far and as wide as I could, things didn't get any better.

If all of the above wasn't enough, I was also in this two-bedded treatment room with an elderly patient who suffered the latter stages of Alzheimer's and thought it was the done thing to keep getting off of her bed, taking her clothes off and parading around the room in the nude. Eventually I was moved to a cubicle on my own, but I think that was purely because by then my mother had arrived and started to have a go at the Doctors about what was happening in this room and how I wasn't well enough to put up with it.

Every doctor asked the same questions, 'How much do you drink?' 'Are you pregnant?'

I tried to be patient but eventually I did let rip and say, 'Look there was no star in the East and my name's not Mary and so I am not pregnant.' During my stay in that hospital I was left in an overflow ward in the A & E department and not a proper ward.

Hygiene was definitely not on the top of the list of that ward… and it seemed it was used until beds were found for people in proper wards, which was supposed to be within a period of 24 hours maximum… I arrived Monday afternoon in the hospital and stayed in this ward Monday night. I was still there by the following Friday. During those days more doctors came and went, more bloody blood tests and still the questions of 'Are you pregnant? How much do you drink?' Hanging above my bed was this big sign 'NIL BY MOUTH'. Every now and again one of the nurses would come and wet my lips with an ice cube to stop them cracking so much. I can remember lying in that ward of six beds, hooked up to drips of saline and bags of intravenous antibiotics, on this bed which was as comfortable as a hospital gurney with a thin mattress thrown on top, not giving a shit whatsoever about what happened in the World Cup, as the match where Beckham got sent off, bellowed from this portable TV that was placed at the end of this room.

By that Friday afternoon I felt so ill, I really was considering making my peace with everyone so that I could fade peacefully into the after-life, but I knew that there was no way I wanted to die in that place... so I discharged myself, and headed for home with bag full of antibiotics. By Sunday morning I couldn't breathe properly, and my husband had to take me back to the hospital. Naturally I got a right old rollicking for discharging myself... but by the sheer luck of a Locum Doctor working on A & E he found exactly why I had Pancreatitis. It was because of my bile duct being blocked with gallstones and I had an inflamed gallbladder. But that was not his main concern. Apparently why I was feeling so ill was because I had Pneumonia as well. Now how the hell can you get pneumonia in hospital without the bloody hospital realising you have such a complaint? Anyway a couple of days under the direction of the Medical Unit (unfortunately back in that A & E Assessment Unit)... they treated the pneumonia and if my chest X-ray was showing no further problems then I could go home on the Tuesday with luck...

On that Tuesday morning my mum came to visit me. I was feeling a hell of a lot better, than the day before, and asked the nurse if it would be OK for me to walk my mum out of the hospital. 'Yes. But before you go let me take out one of those cannulas as you only need one now. But take it easy and when you come back we will take you down for your chest X-ray for the doctor to check when he arrives this afternoon.'

She returned with the necessary item to remove one of the cannulas that was on my left hand. Plastered up and raring to go, mum and I set off along the corridors of the Accident and Emergency Department towards the exit where she was going to call a cab. As we were chatting and giggling like a couple of kids... from the echoes of this corridor came the frantic shouts of, 'Nurse, Nurse quick get a pressure pad.' I looked at mum and said someone's bleeding bad... when all of a sudden my left arm was grabbed and raised high above my head and I was being dragged into this little room and forced to lie down on this examination bed. That person who I thought was bleeding profusely was me…I don't know what happened but the spot where that cannula was removed decided to spray blood up the walls of the corridor and across this crisp white jacket.

Well he stopped the bleeding and padded my hand up and a nurse took me back to the assessment unit… where they said, 'What have you done now?' I never did get to say goodbye to mum properly as once the bleeding was stopped; I was politely informed that I was being taken back to the ward and that I would be OK…and perhaps it was best for her to go home. I knew she had to get back to pick my son up from school. She left a little worried but they reassured her that sometimes this does happen…which did make her feel a little better.

Again I thought, that is it, I won't be going home today. Anyway, the doctor arrived at about 4.30pm, and we chuckled about how I ended up with a hand that was now dressed like a boxer's just before he puts on his glove.

Then came the good news, I could go home... hubby was calling in on his way home from work and was due to turn up at any minute... The doctor wrote out the prescription and the discharge procedure began... Only this time when I told the other half I was allowed home... he checked before he helped me pack up my things.

Again out the door like a bullet out of a gun... And that one experience has made me wary of that hospital. No way do I ever want to be admitted there... fears of what might have been are clearly at the forefront of my mind.

When you are laying there on a bed at the pure mercy of others and they keep asking you basically if you are a 'pregnant alcoholic', your confidence in those professionals plummets. Often in our lifetimes we hear here of horrendous stories about what can happen in hospitals and we just think to ourselves that is bad and move on. It doesn't affect us personally so we don't bat an eyelid really. If we are told of an episode, we comment about how terrible it is… without even thinking about what we would do if we found ourselves in such an awful situation. We walk around oblivious that one day we may be in that same situation… scary.

When the light finally appears at the end of the tunnel and you start to think that you are going to survive, those horrors gradually get swept to the back of our minds. But with me that episode put me in great fear of our local hospital.
From that day on, I swore that should I ever fall ill again, please take me to Darent Valley Hospital, near Dartford…because I am not going to risk ever being put in a position like that ever again by that hospital.

CHAPTER 4 – OCTOBER 2012

People say as long as you have your health you have everything,. Well my health for sure wasn't getting any better, and there was no sign whatsoever of the pain being controlled. I was just living on a cocktail of painkillers (Dihydrocodeine and Paracetamol) along with a daily dosage of Amitriptyline, which was prescribed to me back in 1994 as medical studies into back problems had revealed that these tablets helped people with back problems and eliminated pain.

You read daily in the newspapers about celebrities who end up in rehab because they are hooked on prescription drugs, but when you personally rely on medication to stop your body making it too painful for you to move… then you do begin to see how easy it is to slip into this downward spiral of being hooked on painkillers. And you understand how easily it was for them to get to the point where they now became out of control and irresponsible with their dosages of medication. And you do feel sorry for them, especially if their addiction started because of them wanting pain relief for whatever medical reason they could have.

Well I have never been one of these people who you could call a pill taker… I would prefer to suffer a headache rather than take two paracetamol. But as the years have gone by, all too fast for my liking, as I sit here holding in the bits that wobble and trying my damned hardest to stop everything heading south, I now have to admit that I am finally one of the first people to instead of sitting and suffering in silence, who makes a hasty dash to the medicine chest should I get big toe ache. No I was being a little bit flippant there, toe ache I can endure but back pain and sciatica I can't.

Partly because I am a wimp and don't relish the prospect of lying there in agony until the painkillers kick in and secondly because I know if I don't take something pretty soon this pain is going to get hold of me… and I could well be laid up for days.

Now at this moment in time every bone seemed to ache in my body… yep I had mentally prepared myself for the words Bone Cancer or Multiple Sclerosis. I knew damn well something wasn't right with me… apart from every bone hurting I was gradually losing the grip in my hands, especially if I had to raise my arms above my head to reach for something. The number of things that got knocked off of the shelf and landed either on me or the near the puppies was nobody's business. You can't imagine the pain that a tin of beans falling on your foot can cause.

Having two little puppies, who were just 5 months old, trying to scramble for what I had broken was an unimaginable yet regular occurrence. Apart from having to move the puppies to a safe place till I cleaned up the broken dishes, or the salt that had fallen from the pot, kneeling down was not an option… Thank god for Dyson… yes everything got hoovered up and the floor cleaned until I was certain that there was nothing left around to hurt the pups.

Mind you though I did have to laugh… every time I went to the cupboard they legged it…

I think having things drop on their heads or things that make such a clatter it scared the shite out of them, was just too much … So as I went to the cupboard… the dogs went to their box… I bet they thought it was a hell of a lot safer there than hanging around near me.

What with legs that were giving out, bones aching, my head spinning, every day something happened. One little accident I did have when we had our old dog resulted in me ending up with a couple of broken toes. And that dog soon learned that safety was not at mother's feet but in the dining room.…

And then one day all three happened together… that was it... I stumbled and hey presto there I was with the larder door on me and the doggies thinking they could get in the cupboard and have a rummage and run off with the bottle of Crisp and Dry that was perched on the bottom shelf.

What a mess.… What a bloody palaver that was… trying to wrestle the Crisp and Dry whilst praying to god their little teeth wouldn't pierce the bottle otherwise I would have had two blonde oil slicks running around the house licking each other.

Thank God I have a husband that understands. He just couldn't believe what he came home to that night... a wrecked kitchen. In fact I caused so much damage to the hinge screw holes, he had to take both doors off and turn them so that they opened in the opposite direction.

Hastily I made an appointment with my GP and explained what was happening to me. Never before had I felt as if all my limbs were useless. She told me that the X-rays had shown I had bone spurs in the knees (whatever they were) along with Osteoarthritis. However, her prime concern was something that was showing up in my blood results. Apparently my ESR, (which I later found to mean Erythrocyte Sedimentation Rate) was on the high side, which proved that within this knock kneed knackered old body of mine there was inflammation somewhere.

Next come the 20 questions... you know the ones... Do you smoke? Do you drink? If so, how much alcohol do you drink, and how often? Have you been through the menopause? Has any of your family suffered strokes?

That last question made my ears prick up… because that is what my father died of at the age of 63 back in 1998, and my mother has had several minor strokes commonly known as TIA's (transient ischemic attacks), and added to this list of people who have a history strokes was my Aunt on my mother's side who died at the young age of 49 back in 1967.

Mind you when she mentioned about the smoking… I did have to say to her, 'I have been up and down this Doctor's Surgery more times since I gave up smoking… than I have in the past few years… and they say giving up smoking is healthier for you. Not in my case it seems.'

She sat there and couldn't help but have a chuckle.

All these questions, it was like the Spanish Inquisition. To be honest I don't think they ask you as many questions at Wonga or Match.com when you want to borrow a grand or find a life partner, not that I would know.

When discussing the history of illnesses in the family, diabetes is not one of them, we came across an illness that made my Nan bed-ridden… Rheumatoid Arthritis. A crippling and debilitating illness which over the last few years has made my own mother housebound as well as practically making her infirm… even though she won't admit it.

Immediately an appointment was made for me to see a Rheumatologist at our local hospital in November. Due to the amount of pain I was in… a quick change of medication… out with the Dihydrocodeine and in with the Tramadol. And another load of X-ray forms, this time for my hands and not forgetting the obligatory 'we will make you part with your blood' blood test form.

Finally I was out… thank god for that… after being pulled about, quizzed and told I have something wrong with me as the blood tests indicate inflammation and it must be somewhere in my body… I was finally heading home … ALIVE.

As I crossed the road towards the chemist… for a split second I did contemplate tearing up the prescription and heading straight to the Newsagents next door and buying myself 20 Superking Black.

All this healthy living and giving up smoking was not helping me… so I wondered if that black molten tar that had run through my veins from the age of 16 until I was 52 had blocked all these nasty little things from attacking me. Yes I was suffering with injuries from accidents… but for the last few years nothing else serious had gone wrong with me except for having high blood pressure which was being monitored and treated accordingly, so why has this happened?

Would the Superking cigarettes be the saviour of me… or am I going to have a quick puff, feel sick where I haven't smoked in 2 years and promptly fall to the floor and curl my toes up.

What a bloody option? Die of a stroke through smoking or live and not move… Oh well I suppose I had better cook them dinner…so headed to the chemist instead of the newsagents, and cashed in that prescription.

The chemist looked at me, which we were now on first name terms by, and said 'You are going through it at the moment, aren't you?'

To which I replied, laughingly, 'Yep, the NHS must have seen me coming and liked my company now they can't part with me.'

As he handed the prescription over, my mate behind the counter laughed and said, 'You do know you have to be careful with those tablets as they make you drowsy, so you shouldn't drive or operate machinery?'

'Yep,' I said, 'Does machinery include the oven? Cos if so can you write it on the label? He won't believe me unless there evidence to prove that I am not allowed to touch the cooker.'

No matter what was happening to me and no matter what may be around the corner... deep in my heart I knew that I couldn't afford to lose my sense of humour and neither could I allow this illness to beat me, whatever this illness is. Pain or no pain, I just could not sit there waiting for the day to come when I would die... because believe me, when you can't move and moving your fingers hurts and sends such excruciating pains up your wrists and lower arms… and you can't raise your arms above your shoulders and your legs feel like jelly whilst every muscle hurts in your body… life doesn't feel that good at that particular point in time.

Living with chronic pain is one of the hardest things to bear. We look fine on the outside, we don't have lesions, or coughs, or colds, of any outward symptom that people can see and which show our illness… our symptoms are inside our bodies and just because we look fine, the vast majority of time we are not.

Getting through October, I suppose, was one of the hardest challenges yet. Especially as I had to stop searching for websites, on the internet, that offered you a self diagnosis based on your your symptoms. Another part that I found hard was trying to talk to someone… when you know that something is wrong with you and you don't know what… it is hard to comprehend and you become very anxious, but on the other hand you don't want to sound pathetic or more to the point allow the other person to think you're nothing but a bloody hypochondriac.

Gradually the change of medication helped a little... and helped even more if I took the Tramadol with Paracetamol. But the clumsiness was still there... not being able to open packets, pick money up from the worktop... Even filling the kettle was now a pain... but that problem was solved easily, with a Brita water dispenser for tea and coffee...

A quick trip to Argos and the parting of £70 solved the problem. Now I could make myself a cup of coffee without the fear of having to lift a heavy kettle full of boiling water and dropping it. It wasn't so much for my safety... my greatest fear that an accident would happen, I would drop the kettle and my dogs would get scalded. If that had happened I don't think I could have ever forgiven myself. If I burnt myself ... so be it...but someone else or an animal.... Unforgivable.

As October drew to a close... I still had practically the whole of November to get through before my appointment at the hospital. And my promise of not to self-diagnose my symptoms on the internet to find out what I was suffering from, failed on numerous occasions. Deep down I wished I could have gone to sleep and woke up on the day of my hospital appointment… That will teach me to self-diagnose myself on Google. Christmas was only around the corner, and I didn't seem to have the energy to even think about Christmas yet alone prepare for one. My mind was taken up with the thoughts of what was wrong with me.

CHAPTER 5 – NOVEMBER 2012

Finally, the time had come and the day has arrived for my hospital appointment. The last few weeks seemed to have taken an eternity to get through. Nerves at this precise moment were getting the better of me. What with a rush on at work and only recently changing his job, my hubby couldn't get the time off and my mum was ill herself and unavailable to come with me. I suppose I could have asked a friend or I could've pressed for hubby to have the time off … but I was a big girl. Surely I should be able to go to the hospital on my own? At 54 I don't think I needed anyone to hold my hand, I was not a child but it would have been nice to have the moral support. Lately I am beginning to find that I am losing my confidence in doing things. Perhaps it is because I just under the weather and just need a bit of support now and again.

As the time to my appointment drew even closer my stomach started to churn and I felt a little nauseous, and even though I was showing a brave face on the outside, inside I was scared stiff, I was petrified. My mind was playing repeats, more times that UK Gold does; visions of my Nan lying in bed, crying in pain, not being able to move and being solely dependent on others for her care.

To be lifted from the bed to the commode, as a child I can remember her crying in agony at times. But as a small child, when I was in her room, no matter how much pain she suffered, she endured every second of it, with grace and dignity. I now know by lying next to her frail body my little bones must have hurt her, and I can recall the feel of her arms around me with her twisted hands cradling me. The fear of ending up like that petrifies me. I don't want to be infirm… I don't want to have to rely on others for care. I don't want to lose my independence.

I know medical science has progressed greatly since the early 1960's but still today Rheumatoid Arthritis scares me to death. Here I was in my mid 50's waking up feeling like a 90 year, full of aches and pains.

In the mornings if I did manage to get some decent sleep I would wake as stiff as a board... unbendable and definitely not pliable. If I knew I had to be somewhere for an early morning appointment, like today at the hospital, I would have to get up at the crack of dawn in order to have enough time for my body to un-stiffen and limber up... in order for my joints to move more freely.

As I arrived at the hospital, the fear was increasing... I hate hospitals at the best of times and that is when other people are the patients... When I am the patient you can well imagine how scared I get. Especially after my terrible hospital experience of thinking I was going to die back in 1998.

By luck I wasn't sat there waiting too long before the nurse called me in to do the preliminary examination. You know the one. The one where she checks your height, your weight (and you know the scales are going to say one at a time please) and your blood pressure and of course the urine test... whilst not forgetting to ask the Spanish Inquisition questions all over again. Do you smoke? Do you drink? So on and so on. Now I am getting good at this... I can even pre-empt the answer before they finish the question.

Practice makes perfect as they say... or could it be that I have heard these same damn questions so many bloody times, that the answers are imprinted on my brain, that my mouth automatically responds, without me even putting any effort into it.

Then we arrived at the worst part of this preliminary health checkup... a form. My god, holding a pen was now a thing of the past. As soon as I applied pressure to the pen, my thumb and forefinger would tell my brain, 'Hey stop that I hurt'. Which usually ended with me grasping my thumb which was in agony and saying, 'That bloody well hurt.'

I felt guilty not being able to do it, but the nurse understood and told me that she would go through the form with me when I went in to see the Doctor. Knowing that little bit of help was going to come seemed to fractionally lighten the burden of guilt I had started to carry around with me.

The burden of guilt, if I can make you understand, started off bum-bag size but as things got broken, things were not done in the household chores department, etc, etc, etc. This little bum-bag was now over spilling into a hand-bag full of guilt which had even started to over spill into a suitcase that would have been classed as 'excess baggage' by Ryan Air.

Silly little things were now turning into major issues. Apart from aching I was fatigued... I wanted to sleep yet couldn't. Every large muscle was aching along with practically every bone in my body.

Every day was now becoming a struggle in one way or another. I was either too tired to do anything or I ached too much. I had so many questions I wanted to ask this consultant but I knew until he had seen me and did tests, he was as much in the dark as to the reason why I felt like this and what could be wrong as I was.

In the waiting room I looked around and saw that there were people of my age, and one person looked even younger than me, sitting there waiting to see the Rheumatologist. Somehow that offered comfort, perhaps knowing that I wasn't the only one going through such hard times, health wise, didn't make me feel so alone.

Sitting there, waiting, I got chatting to another woman, near my age, I would say, and she was suffering the same. Every bone, every muscle ached... morning, noon and night. They too thought she could have Rheumatoid Arthritis and she told me of her fears of being bed-ridden. We were just chatting to each other, and somehow, even though we didn't know one another from Adam, we started to feel as if we were not entirely alone and feeling as if we were battling something that some people don't and won't even try to understand.

Then the nurse called my name. In I went and the Rheumatologist asked the questions on the form and filled in the answers for me... I was so grateful, that I could have got up and kissed him. Next he took a look at my hand X-rays and said that he could see wear-and-tear and what looks like joint erosion as well as effusion of the joints... (Whatever that is, when its at home.)

The only way to confirm how much erosion and effusion there was in my hands would be to order an MRI scan on both of my hands, which he did. He immediately wrote and signed the appropriate form out requesting the scan. Until my next visit, he decided to prescribe me with Arcoxia 90mg tablets, which is an anti-inflammatory drug. Straight away I had to tell him that, I have had problems in the past with regards anti-inflammatory drugs and how they caused me to have upset stomachs.

'No fear', he replied 'These can be taken on an empty stomach.'

I immediately thought thank God for that… maybe now some of this inflammation will subside. Next I was given another form for a bloody test to check my Rheumatoid Factor, and again to check my ESR levels as they were elevated.

One of the suggestions he gave me was the option of physiotherapy, for my knees. Learning to use the quadriceps in your legs helps to keep the knee injury free and more flexible. I didn't care what it did; I would try anything to stop some of these aches and pains. So I snapped his arms off and agreed to see the physiotherapist. Yet another form was signed which I was told that I had to hand in to the Physiotherapy Department, located at the entrance to the left of the main building, on my way out of the hospital.

He told me that he couldn't give me a timeframe for a follow up appointment as he didn't know the waiting times for MRI Scans but he assured me that as soon as I had the scans the hospital would be in touch with me to make an appointment for me to see him.

So armed with blood test forms, MRI Scan forms, a Physiotherapist letter plus another prescription for another pill for me to pop I left that consulting room a little happier but still none the wiser. I suppose on my first visit it was too much for me to expect him to say… you have this and you need to take this and do that. I suppose deep down that is what I was hoping for but knew would never happen.

November was turning out to be no better than October really… even though I was now under the hospital and it might only be just a matter of time before I would be sorted and back to having virtual pain-free days, other than the little niggles in my back, these last two months had taken their toll on me.

It had been a real emotional rollercoaster. As I got off the bus heading towards the chemist… I just hoped and prayed that these tablets would remove that inflammation, and I could start to feel as normal as possible… for a woman of my age.

CHAPTER 6 – DECEMBER 2012

December arrived, and still no news of any dates for my MRI Scan. When you don't feel well, and you want to know what is wrong with you, you will the postman to deliver you a letter so that you know you have a)not been forgotten by the NHS and b) that you don't have too long to wait before you find out what is making you so unwell.

Here we are in December and not a thing planned for Christmas. I know I am not the most organized person at Christmas but I am better than this. The thought of bringing a Christmas together was panicking me in a way… Something I never used to suffer from… I would take things in my stride, deal with them, and promptly move on to the next problem.

But lately the simplest little thing bugged me… my patience was worn out with everyone and everything. Even the dogs and their puppy ways was beginning to get to me.

I had been stabbed with needles, prodded, poked, questioned and maneuvered into positions my body didn't even know existed, and still here we were over 2 months down the line with not knowing why I was feeling this way.

I had only been on the Arcoxia a couple of weeks, and it was helping but my hopes of it being the wonder drug were slowly day by day getting trashed. It managed to relieve some pain but it never relieved it all.

Eventually I received the letter from the MRI Department and my scan was book for Saturday 5th December 2013 at 5pm at Medway Hospital.

The thought that things were going to get moving after Christmas cheered me up a little, but there was still Christmas to get through.

But hubby, bless him, said that he would cook the dinner, and he would write the Christmas cards as I was still finding it hard to write and hold a pen.. Holding a pen made my thumb and forefinger ache like crazy as well as making the muscle in the top of my right arm go into spasm.

We used the internet to order the vast majority of Christmas presents, and the love of my life, wrapped them. This year there were more presents to wrap, as we were blessed with a new arrival to our family, in early December.

About 7 days before Christmas I received a letter through the post from my GP. They wanted me to call the surgery and book a telephone consultation. They had received the X-ray results and wanted to discuss them with me. The doctor spoke to me the following day or the day after, I can't quite remember now, but she said by the looks of the X-rays I might have signs of Osteoporosis.

Talk about a downer… how much more can go wrong?

Just before Christmas Eve I was phoned by the physiotherapy department and they asked me to attend a consultation on the 2nd January 2013. Note made on calendar and I was determined not to allow whatever was wrong with me spoil Christmas.

It was only on Christmas morning that he finally realized that he had actually wrapped his own Christmas presents… we did laugh about that. And he said, 'Don't worry, I will act all surprised.' True to his word he cooked the diner without too many hitches and without too much pain, Christmas came and Christmas went… I wasn't feeling better by vast amounts, if anything it would only be slightly. I still had no energy and felt totally fatigued but if anything the pain was not as severe.

Roll on 2013…

CHAPTER 7 – JANUARY 2013

New Year came and went, in fact I was glad to get the decorations down a day earlier. When you are not well, to put it bluntly you just can't be arsed with Christmas, presents, and all the paraphernalia of being cheerful, whilst super-gluing a fake smile to your fizzog (face). But in true stiff-upper-lip Brit fashion… a fake smile was there, a warm Christmas cheer along with the face-paint that is put on double thick to hide those bags that have taken up permanent residence under your eyes.

Mind you when the Christmas guests all left that was it… face-off, the shoes were kicked off straight away and there I was curled up nice and cosy on the settee all ready for a good kip, which didn't take long to happen. I think as soon as my head hit that pillow on Christmas Day I was out like a light.

It was now the 2nd of January and the second day of a new year and here I was heading back for the hospital to be manipulated once again.

This time I didn't have the trek there... hubby was still on Xmas leave and so I was chauffeured to the hospital. By luck, parking was no problem. I don't know about any of you and your hospitals but you can queue half way round Gillingham in a traffic jam, waiting to get parked near that hospital at times.

It was freezing in that hospital... but it wasn't long before I was called...thankfully.

The physiotherapist was lovely...she explained about what she did and I was not to be worried about asking her questions and even if she didn't know the answer, she would find out and get back to me. She made me feel quite at ease. We went through why I was there and she had to stop me when I started to ask about what she could for my hands, neck (which had now decided to ache in sympathy) and shoulders.

Unfortunately, she could only deal with my knee problems. But she did say that I could contact my consultant and get another referral. One of the things she could do for me was to offer me a place on the *Escape New Pain Course*, which they held at local health centre's around Medway, which I agreed to.

Upon examination she found I had a vast amount of muscle weakness in my legs and she only wanted me to do the first couple of exercises that were on a printed sheet. She explained that due to how bad my legs were, that doing too much could be bad for them and it was now down to finding the right balance of exercise, so that I didn't cause more damage than there already was. The balance needed for me to gain muscle strength without paining the muscles too much. So her recommendation was small steps with regards to exercise at this moment in time and that was probably the best way to go for now, until I had garnered enough strength in the muscles to proceed onto the next stage.

After lying on this bed, in her little consulting cubicle, for 20 minutes doing these exercises, my thighs couldn't take any more… It didn't feel like a pain you get when you over exercise, this felt like an ache almost immediately and the pain seemed to intensify the more I did. Mind you I know I shouldn't have but when she left the cubicle to sort out the Escape Knee Pain Class I was glad of a breather… Just like a child, not wanting to be caught by the teacher, for slacking, there I was lying on this bed listening to see if I could hear her coming.

Finally, the session over, thank God and the next appointment booked for the end of January. Hubby had waited for me so we left the hospital and headed straight for home. Brrrr… That bracing wind was very cold that day. We were glad to get back into the warm.

Three more days to go and I'd once again be back up at that very same hospital, only this time having my hands MRI scanned. What joys being ill can bring?

Saturday arrived and I got ready to go again… only this time to the MRI suite to be scanned… my God I sound like a pack peas on the conveyor belt at Tesco's. Being shut in small confined spaces is something I don't like. I can't say I am claustrophobic, but I just don't like small closed-in spaces.

The thought of going through that MRI scanner was really putting the heebie-jeebies up me. I can tell you that.

Letters come through the door and I read them, but sometimes I do forget what they say… I completely missed the bit that no jewellery whatsoever is to be worn or make up. Anyway at 5pm on a Saturday evening we arrived at the MRI suite in plenty of time for me to be scanned. Booking in was no problem. The first problem was the jewellery I was wearing. It all had to be all removed and luckily my husband was there and he looked after my rings, necklaces, and earrings. I quickly went to the ladies and got most of the slap off of my face. The other problem that threw itself at us was with the MRI equipment being used that day.

To cut a long story short, the scanner in the MRI Suite had broken down and they had a replacement scanner parked outside the hospital. The backlog in the MRI suite, with regards to keeping to appointment times, was due to the replacement scanner in the car park breaking down and them having to wait for another scanner to arrive. We didn't wait too long before they called me in and said that I would be having my scan done in the replacement scanner in the car park. No problems as far as I was concerned, this sooner this was over the better. A lovely nurse walked me around to this trailer, which held the scanner and once the scan was over I could return to the MRI unit.

Fine… don't care where they do it, but hurry up and do it, because I am getting nervous here and if I get too nervous you will be scanning me, in between my visits to the ladies to spend a penny. I suppose that is 20p now due to inflation…oh the good old Tories… don't you love their cries of we're all in this together lark… No we are in this shite and the Tories are there on the other side watching you struggle.

Just as I walked to the scanner, the nurse explained what they wanted me to do…they wanted me to lay down on the bed, on my stomach, with my arm stretched out above my head whilst my hand was placed in this contraption, so that the MRI scanner could do its work. She said the first scan takes about 30 minutes, what with getting you prepared and getting the machine lined up etc.

Immediately I thought to myself, FGS I can't lift my arm above my shoulder now without it hurting like crazy and now you want me to be bloody Superman...

Finally we reached the scanning vehicle. You know what those refrigerated lorries look it as they chug away...well this is exactly what that scanner looked like... panic set in believe me... and it took all my will to remain calm and climb the metal stairs into the trailer and not run (as if I could) for the hills.

I got undressed... into the gown and then upon this table, padded up, headphones on to drown out the noise of the scanner, a buzzer placed in my free hand, for me to press if I got panicky, whilst my right hand was clasped firmly in the special case, my heart was pounding so hard and so fast I thought any minute now I am going to have a bloody heart attack... The hole that my hand and I were supposed to have fitted through seemed no bigger than the hole in a

Polo…more and more the claustrophobia started to set in.

'Deep breaths girl you can do this,' I thought to myself whilst in my mind I had visions of being stuck in this machine and never getting out and when the table started to play up… those visions were now turning into nightmares, my heart was racing so fast I felt physically sick at one point...

Time after time they tried to get the table to load into the scanner, but it was having none of it. They did stay that it played up earlier but a computer reset sorted the problem. She would do this reset again… so off of the table I was taken, back into the nurse's area whilst they ran a diagnostic test and did yet another computer reset.

Every bit of me just wanted to get dressed and get out of trailer and head for home.

Again they tried, but no this machine was not having any of it… no way was this scan going to take place… and as the nurse pushed and pulled the table to make it work, the more the blood drained from my face, because I now had the fear that this machine will allow me to go in and not let me out.

The poor nurse must have seen the blood drain from my face and she reassured me that, they could easily pull the table out if needed. I thought to myself…'yep fine chance, if you can't push it in, it's not going to let you pull it out now is it.'

Eventually time was called and they said the machine was not going to reset properly and they sent me back, after getting dressed, to the main MRI Suite.

When I arrived back there…I was then informed, they had no spare time to do my MRI Scan that day and could I return Thursday at 10am when they would guarantee it would be done.

Hubby was not happy, but to be honest, I don't think he would have chanced going through that thing if he had seen the palaver of trying to get it going.

Thursday came… quicker than I wanted to be honest. Anyway off to the hospital one more time, minus the make-up and jewellery … and back to the MRI Suite all ready for my claustrophobic hour with a machine that I was sure had it in for me.

When I was called, the machine I was about to be scanned by…was bigger and seemed to have a larger hole than the one the Saturday before… not much but larger all the same. Bloody hell I thought, I hope I get done this time.

Undressed and all gowned up, I was laid on the table… my arm once again stretched out so far that the pain in my shoulder at times brought tears to my eyes. After going through the rigmarole of having the headphones on and the buzzer in my spare hand, the machine finally started to chug and churn and do its job. It even roared, and it rattled like crazy with its magnets at one point. Lying there in this one position, I just kept thinking and wondering how much longer I had to be in this painful position. After about 25 minutes I was removed from the scanner… the clinician saw how much agony I was in with my shoulder and offered to do the other hand another day.

I wanted this over and done with. So I told her to carry on and get the other hand scanned…which she did. Luckily this time, the scan didn't take so long and it wasn't long before I was removed from that wretched machine once and for all.

I was told the results would be sent to my consultant and I will hear from the Rheumatology Department as to when my next appointment would be.

MRI over with… thank God. Shoulders and upper arms aching well now, and my right arm feels like jelly, on well my new perfume, Eau de Deep Heat will soon ease those pains…

Finally I got indoors to find a letter laying on the doormat saying that my Escape Knee Pain 5 Week Course starts on the 28th January 2013 at a health centre in Rochester.

It was soon Monday the 28th January 2013 and my first day at the Escape Knee Pain 5 Week Course. The class started at 9.30 am, so I was to be up long before then, in order to limber up enough to be able to make it. Gone are the days, when I could jump out of bed, rush around like a headless chicken and be out of the door in 30 minutes… with hair and makeup done. Now it is a matter of taking things dead slow until I can limber up this old body enough to muster the first move yet alone anything else.

Oh the grand old joys of getting old.

I arrived at the centre well in time; where I met up with 4 more ladies who were on the course as well as two gentlemen. Mind you the men only turned up the first week.

They physiotherapists who ran the group were helpful, encouraging and would answer any questions you had... but then came the part called exercise time... oh my God doing simple exercises really started to hurt, in fact as the 5 weeks progressed the pain was more and more.

I was beginning to get to the stage where I knew I would not be able to move for a couple of days after, what with all this exercise. And to make matters worse, the following day, the 29th, I had to go back to Medway hospital to see the physiotherapist there. How the hell was I going to mange?

I could see the benefit of those exercises and to be honest whilst on the course I took the attitude of *No Pain No Gain*. Which now I know is and was the completely wrong attitude to take when you suffer from Polymyalgia Rheumatica.

By luck I had been on the Arcoxia 2 months or more and even though they didn't take the pain away fully, I think they helped and they took the edge off the pain off but they certainly didn't make me pain-free.

But now, this whole illness and what it does to your body was getting to me… I was fed up with feeling like shite. I was fed up with aching all over and above all stinking of Eau de Deep Heat and rattling when I walked, due to the amount of pills I was popping down my throat.

And if the aches and pains were not enough to make you sink into the depths of despair, the constant fatigue surely was. I had been tired in my life before …but this… I'd never known anything like it. All I can say is that it was really debilitating.

The following morning, full of aches and pains, I attended the hospital once again for my Physiotherapy appointment… and another session of exercise. Now that I was on the course, the physiotherapist said that she didn't need to see me at the hospital anymore and would wait to see how I got on and whether the therapists at the Knee Pain Classes thought I should have more therapy.

Two days of exercise… after just getting rid of the pains of having that MRI…did me in for January. Roll on February; things couldn't get any worse… surely?

CHAPTER 8 – MARCH 2013

February came and February went… with not much happening other than my visits to the 'Escape Knee Pain Classes', where I think the physiotherapists could work out why my muscles were aching so much when others in the class were getting increased strength in theirs.

I explained to them that no matter how much I tried, I collapsed in agony with my thigh muscles feeling as if they are just about to pop out of my leg. They felt so tense and so tender to touch. Finally they told me to tell my consultant… at my next visit set for the 13th of this Month.

I still attended the glasses but I was getting no better, in fact my legs ache even more after the exercise session.

Finally, it is the 13th March 2013 and I'll get to hear some of the results. How long has this been going on… since November 2012 and still the consultant hasn't told me what is wrong? Hopefully today will be the day.

One good thing now is that the hospital have been sending me copies of letters sent to my GP and my MRI scan showed that were was effusion in the joints in both of my hands at the 1st, 2nd, 3rd and 4th metacarpophalangeal joints as well as the 1st carpometacarpal (CMC) joint on my right hand. The left hand also revealed degenerative changes to the 1st carpometacarpal (CMC) joint…

Google is your friend at times. Just searching Google told me exactly what was happening to my hands. When I told my husband I had to laugh when he said, 'So your hands are fucked, then.' Which made me burst into laughter as this is his favourite saying when something breaks… he just looks at you and says, in such a dry manner, 'That's fucked.'

At times I think his humour has been the only thing that has kept me going… and got me through some of the darkest days.

So there I am sitting there and waiting patiently for the nurse to call my name… I don't know what it was but something inside of me… just knew he was going to say something that I would be totally unprepared for.

Then they called my name... he went through the MRI scan and told me what they can do for my hands in the future. But his concern was primarily once again... my ESR levels had not really reduced that much since being put on the Arcoxia.

Rheumatoid arthritis, luckily, was ruled out, as the rheumatoid factor test came back negative. That was it... if it is not Rheumatoid arthritis... is it Bone Cancer... the fear was welling up in me now... Then he fired another load of questions off and asked me to stand up and try to raise my arms... it hurt... then he felt the muscles in both of my upper arms and I could have screamed out in agony... they were so tender. He then asked how long it took me to get myself limbered up after getting up stiff. When I told him it could range from between 45 mins to a couple of hours... he then diagnosed Polymyalgia Rheumatica and decided to put me on a course of steroids.

What is this disease, I have never heard of it? But he gave me a prescription for steroids. I started at a course of 20mg Prednisolone and instructions how to decrease it over the course of the next three months and I was to go back to see him in 3 months.

Steroids, please don't say these are going to make me look like a sumo wrestler, but a quick search on the internet put my mind at rest that the steroids I was now prescribed were not anabolic kind.

I was so shell-shocked that I left his office, in such a daze that I left the prescription on his desk… and really didn't have my mind on anything…other than to read the leaflets he gave me about this disease. He told me that it is controllable and some people do recover… however there is a great chance that at some point I might have a flare-up and will have to go through all of the trials and tribulations of sorting the medication out all over again.

Thank God for that nurse, who came running after me, and giving me the prescription… I would have wandered out of that hospital quite easily without giving the prescription a second thought.

Along with the leaflets were the usual blood test forms, which have to be done every 2 months, primarily to check my ESR and CPR (C-reactive protein) levels as well as liver function and full blood count.

I booked my next consultation appointment for July 2013. Getting my head around all this was taking its time. I just couldn't come to terms with what was going on in my body. The more I searched Google the more I was learning. It seems there are a lot of people diagnosed with this and there are stories of people who are having a really rough time.

One thing the leaflet did mention is this...

Giant Cell Arteritis

PMR is sometimes associated with painful inflammation of the arteries of the skull. This is called giant cell arteritis (GCA) or temporal arteritis and needs prompt treatment as there's a risk of damage to the arteries of the eye. About 20% of PMR patients also develop GCA, while 40-60% of patients with GCA have symptoms of PMR.

The symptoms of GCA are:

- *Severe headaches and pain in the muscles of the head*
- *Tenderness at the temples*
- *Pain in the jaw, tongue or side of the face when chewing*
- *Pain and swelling in the scalp*
- *Blurred or double vision*

Great, so things could go from bad to worse... and with my luck so far... that list of 20% of patients they refer to in that leaflet is bound to have my name on it.

Watch out Google... here I come again... I want to know everything about this bloody disease and it seems that the only way to treat it is to bugger up your immune system... And the worst part of is this, should I come into contact with someone with shingles of chicken pox I have to go to my GP immediately and get treatment... FGS what do you do? Do you shout could all chicken pox or shingles please raise your hands as you step onto the bus? Do you avoid every child and look at every person in Morrison's or Tesco's to see if they look a little ill… and if so do you go up and ask them… whether they have chicken pox or shingles?

Can you just imagine it though? Walking up the tin can aisle and then some plucky person steps in front of you as you are just about to grab that tin of garden peas, what do you do? Do you ask them if it is bad acne and if so direct them to the aisle with those medicated face washes or abandon your trolley, run from the store and get to the GP's as quick as you can, if they reply shingles or chicken pox?

The very day after my consultation, I started this Prednisolone… 20 mg and what a life change I had to make. I was sure it would send my whole body into shock.

All of my adult life I have never been able to get up and eat… the thought of downing a bowl of porridge or Frosties makes me want to literally be sick… its only after I have been up a few hours and several cups of coffee later then I can eat but first thing in the morning… yuck.

When you are dieting you are told skimmed milk, no fat is the best for you... no fat and is healthier... now that I was taking Prednisolone it was advised, and I can't remember who by, but it could have only been the GP or Consultant, to drink semi-skimmed milk.

I love milk in my coffee but seriously to drink a glass of milk is another thing that makes me want to heave. But I suppose if I have to drink this stuff, I must. Your whole life starts to change... apart from feeling downright ill at times, your routine, your diet and even skincare changes. Nothing is ever the same again. That is when the depression starts to set-in. When you are on your own and you have time to think.

When your immune system is being shot to shreds, you are susceptible to catching whatever goes around. During this month, I caught a cold... it was well into April before I finally managed to kick it. Yes I am one that might get a stingy throat and a sniffle but never do these two symptoms turn into a full blown cold. This one did though... and to be perfectly honest it knocked me for six, I was hacking and coughing and sneezing and spluttering for at least 3 weeks... unbelievable! The others in my house caught the cold, and within a week it was gone... In fact, during the whole time I was sneezing and spluttering, they caught the bloody cold, got over it and were back to full health.

One of the side-effects of Prednisolone apparently is Osteoporosis... brilliant here we go, didn't my GP say that I could have that when my hands were X-rayed? Yes she did Oh well at least if I am in permanent plaster cast, I won't break anything... one consolation I suppose. There again, if invited to a party that has a film theme to it, I could wrap a few bandages around myself...and hey presto I have the perfect fancy dress costume... the mummy.

My next appointment at the hospital was booked for July. And the consultant gave me the forms for another blood test to be carried out – another stab-and-prick-until-you-find-blood session – which he wanted done just before my next appointment with him.

I followed his instructions carefully, and to the letter… I was starting to feel better… brilliant … great I have kicked this…. Or so I thought.

CHAPTER 9 – JULY 2013

The last three months, had been up and down… the lower the dosage I took of this Prednisolone, the more I started to ache. I just couldn't believe it… I thought I was doing fine and kicking butt out of this PMR but alas no, it seemed as if my body just didn't want to part with this bloody Polymyalgia Rheumatica.

When your muscles ache constantly, and you have no strength or stamina, doing the easiest of tasks feels like you have just decided to do the London Marathon… How some of those athletes collapse after they have run over 26 miles is just how you feel when you have just mopped the kitchen floor.

I knew with my back problems, there were times when I couldn't do things, and had to take things at a slow pace… but that was purely to stop niggling pains turning into ferocious attacks of sciatica. I learnt to pace myself, judge things and cope with life. But lately, I can't even make arrangements for the next day because I don't know how I will feel. Gradually as the Prednisolone is being decreased the more days I am having of rolling out of the bed and straight into the recliner.

During the last three months my GP has called me back to check my blood pressure and found that it has increased and he has again altered my blood pressure medication.

Blood pressure, PMR, colds, flu, and fear of chicken pox… am I ever going to be ME ever again? Me, the person who could cope with bad backs and sciatica and the problems they caused with sleepless nights yet still managed to have some quality of life. I couldn't walk far but that didn't stop me going out. Places we visited used to have plenty of benches to sit down on so that my back got a rest but lately it has been literally sit down, move to next bench, sit down yet again and rest and then onto the next bench.. The fatigue and lack of stamina are increasing… I don't like this at all and will be glad when I go back to the hospital… To be perfectly honest I think I was feeling a whole lot better before I ever went to the hospital.

Don't tell me this is going to turn out to be yet another NHS hospital mayhem, cock-up, or blunder, whichever you want to call it; only this time it is me who is at the centre of the NHS nightmare? Only this would be my second fiasco... please no!

Finally the day arrived for my consultation... and when I arrived at the Rheumatology department it was jammed pack. I mean there was not a seat in the house at all... people were standing there in the waiting area... and all you could hear was moan, moan, and bloody moan.

Mind you I couldn't blame them, because apparently the hospital administrators had double booked the patients that day. Whether it was to clear a back-log or an administrative error I don't know. But that hospital waiting room was jammed pack with patients. By luck, my consultant was not double booked and was running a delay of only 15 mins... unlike those other poor sods standing around and waiting; their delay was along the lines of 1½ hours.

Eventually my name was called and I was ushered in again to see the consultant. I walked into the room and he was reading my blood test results. Yes as he looked at my ESR and C-reactive Protein readings, he shrugged and you could see him contemplating what to do. Finally he looked up and spoke, 'Your blood test results are not good, there is no decrease in readings in fact they are higher. I want to try you on this drug named Methotrexate, at a weekly dose of 15mg and 5 mg of Folic Acid, 24 hours later.'

And then news I really didn't want to hear. I was politely informed it is one of the drugs that they use in Polymyalgia Rheumatica treatment to treat this disease and it has some side effects and as from now I would need blood tests carried out every two months and here is a leaflet to read… about the side effects… and how the drug works… This drug by all accounts attacks the immune system and can take up to 12 weeks before it starts working and I won't feel any benefit until about 3 months time. What he wanted to do is to get me on this drug and off of the steroids as soon as was feasibly possible. Which I suppose is understandable.

I was given a form to take to X-ray to have my chest X-rayed as Methotrexate can cause breathlessness and have an impact on your lungs. Great… why don't you attack another organ… if I'm not tired enough now there is a chance I will be a breathless, fatigued, knock kneed, knackered, old nosebag… brilliant.

The shock of what was said in that consultation about the new drug and what it is used primarily for and why they are giving it to me seemed such a haze…Nothing was sinking in. My mind was awash with words and the word that kept coming into my brain was Methotrexate, simply because whilst sitting waiting for my X-ray I kept reading the side effects of this drug, and had heard of this drug before when someone I knew was being treated for cancer. There I was sitting in this waiting room to nuked, not knowing a thing and having a sense of panic invade my body like I have never experienced before. I felt alone, my mind was racing, weird thoughts were entering my head and that bloody word cancer kept springing up in my mind... FFS it's not cancer it's Polymyalgia Rheumatica... brain please get a grip of yourself.

My name was called and X-ray done and I was told that the results would be with my consultant within 10 days and he would contact me if there are any problems. Well I didn't hear anything so it must have been OK.

Armed yet again with more bloody forms for blood test butchering and a pink form to hand in at the Out-Patients Booking Desk for an appointment to be me made for me in October 2013, I walked totally oblivious and like a zombie straight passed the booking desk holding my pink form in one hand and my bus ticket in the other.

Even the warm air of that day, didn't seem to have any heat in it...and I got on the bus, showed my ticket, sat on my seat and was half way down Chatham Hill before I looked down and realised I still had the pink appointment form in my hand. Bollox. What do I do now? Do I get off the bus at the Town Centre hop back on another one, go back to the hospital make the appointment or go home and phone the consultants secretary and explain and see if she can book me in. There was no great debate…home I came and phoned the hospital and the secretary was very understanding and made my appointment and said a letter will be send in the post.

To be honest I think this was the time when the darkest thoughts of having this illness started to enter my mind. Especially after I read about the dangers of this drug and how you can even lose your hair. Here I was now at the age of 56 not knowing what the future held at all.

I started taking this drug after the weekend… I didn't want to take it before the weekend, just in case it had an immediate effect and I was groggy over the weekend. One thing that I do know, right from a child, drugs would invariably upset my stomach.

It took a hell of a lot of trial and error to find the right blood pressure tablet… so putting me on a drug that was so strong (and as my GP called it dangerous if not monitored) didn't enthrall me at all.

Then came the sore mouth, and the upset stomachs… but I persevered, thinking that with each dose my body would get used to it. The prospect of spending half of my life now in the loo was not a prospect I wanted but it was something that I having to endure.

When drugs upset you so much, you develop a fear of going out, just in case… your sat nav tells you where to park, but it doesn't tell you where the nearest toilet is. If you want to visit parks, pubs, and places of interest, TomTom's your man, but if you want a bog in an emergency… TomTom is not so obliging. So unless you know the place where you are going then you develop this fear of what am I going to do… if I can't find a loo?

Its OK to keep dishing out pills but for the person who has to keep taking them… a little more consideration should be given… hint for you there TomTom.

Every week as I took this drug I prayed that my symptoms would subside… they never did… if anything they just got worse… and then the depression started to set in and I was becoming more and more irritable. It only took the slightest little thing to happen for me to start ranting and raving... I felt deep down I was getting to the point where I didn't care if I lived or died. The aches and pains were there... in my shoulders, arms, thighs, hips, hands, back and neck. Even my Eau de Deep Heat was not having much of an impact now. Too tired to do this, and if I managed to do anything... I was getting out of breath pretty soon.

I know I couldn't walk far before my back ached... but a quick sit down and a gentle mooch would solve that problem. Now it was if everything was aching. Before this really took hold of me, my hubby and I would go out and photograph places. Yes he knew I couldn't climb mountains and I needed a lot of rest-breaks but we did manage to get out and about.

Not now though... I am too tired, too fatigued or too scared to leave the loo. This is not life this is a bloody existence. It was affecting my life in such a way, even the hobbies that we loved were now in jeopardy.

I knew I had to dig deep inside of me… somewhere in there was some fight left… yes it was going to hurt, yes it was going to be bloody hard work just mustering up the energy but was going to hurt whether I stayed at home or go out.

With Imodium taken at times, just in case one of those nasty side-effects decided to rear its ugly head, we went to some places, mainly coastal places, where we knew there would be plenty of seating areas and places where we knew we didn't have to park far, far away.

If we did have had luck and couldn't find a car park near the front, slowly we would stroll, take our photographs, sit down on a bench and have a coffee and then when the time arrived to go home, he would get the car, drive down to where I was and I would get back in.

Who knows, it has only been a few of doses of these tablets, things might settle down and I could be well on the road to recovery.

I can't say it enough. This PMR is a funny old thing… there are days when you just want to sit there and do absolutely nothing and then you get a couple of good days, where the niggles are there but you feel better… only trouble is at times those good moments are short-lived.

In a few weeks time my husband is taking his annual leave. We know we can't go far with the dogs but we want to go out for days, all I am hoping and praying for at the moment is that I will be OK.

Think positive… think ahead and above all try to stay bloody sane.

CHAPTER 10 – THE LAST FIVE MONTHS OF 2013

The last five months of 2013 have been nothing but a bloody struggle to be perfectly honest. I was doing as ordered taking this Methotrexate and lowering the steroids as told to by the hospital... but there were no signs of improvement... There isn't a day that goes by where something doesn't hurt. Or a week that goes by where I am fully confident of being away from the house just in case the medication decides to send me on a marathon to and from the toilet.

What with countless blood tests that leave me with a badly bruised arm and bruises now starting to appear everywhere on me... to the point that I really do look like a battered wife... The dog treads on my foot... I'm bruised. I knock my hand on something... I'm bruised. Even if I go to put something on and catch my arm ... I'm bruised.

According to the medication this is one of the side effects and if there is excessive unexplained bruising then you should report it… as for my bruising I know what causes it…bumping into things, knocking things… every bruise that is on my body I know exactly how it got there.

Back in October I went for my next consultation up the hospital… and yet again the ESR and C-reactive Protein readings were elevated… they were not going down … they were increasing if anything. Looking back on the results I think these readings were lower before I started on the steroids and all subsequent drugs that followed.

During one of my other consultations, I asked the consultant if I will ever be cured… he gave me hope and said yes. According to him it was just a matter of time and finding the right things to treat it. The consultant then decided to increase the Methotrexate, from 15mg to 20mg for four weeks and then up to 25mg until the next consultation in two months.

Walking out of that hospital, I had never felt so low… I wanted to cry and I felt downright ill. I managed to get home and as I walked indoors the tears just fell... There was no stopping them, it was as if floodgates had finally been opened and every pent up feeling, emotion and anxiety was trying to escape from my body through my tears.

When I looked in the mirror a shadow of my former self stared back at me... my hair was limp, dull, with no shine or sheen whatsoever to it; by luck though, I wasn't losing it... I suppose that is one advantage. My face was puffy due to the steroids. My skin was broken out in spots that had not just gone away, but turned to small scabs and were taking an eternity to heal. The tears flowed once more... which didn't help my appearance...

Bad hair days were common and even a trip to the hairdressers didn't have much of an impact... because no matter what she tried to do, there was no more volume in my hair and it had completely lost its bounce. So I knew as I sat there crying a hair make-over won't even make me feel better... and will be just a waste of money.

Gone were the days when you occasionally had a bad hair, which was usually one or two a month... good hairs were the ones you thought of now; when am I getting a good hair day? And you wrote them on the calendar because they are so few and far between, that you had to celebrate their anniversary.

And the thought of having to increase this medication just sent shivers down my spine and caused me to panic inside. Since taking it July 2013, one of the side effects I did get was a sore mouth... ulcers, even blisters and spots appearing on my tongue... At times it was painful to eat... so ice-cube remedy it was. Suck on an ice-cube until it numbs your mouth... that worked for a while but my immune system was now shot away... if I now had one.

Still I did as I was told and increased the next dose and the one after that and maybe the third, but things were getting no better... If anything again they were getting worse. I had been back to my GP to discuss my medications and left there feeling as despondent as could be as they told me that Polymyalgia Rheumatica is controlled not cured. There is always that chance that there will be a relapse or a flare-up of the symptoms. I just felt as if I was finally on the scrap heap... just jostling my position in the queue and waiting for the day to come when they take me out in my box.

In front of people I acted cheerfully as if nothing was bothering me... but deep inside of me I just wanted to kick shite out of something or someone... I felt bitter, twisted and at breaking point. How much more I have got to endure... before there is a glimmer of light? I knew we were just around the corner again from Christmas... and the prospect of facing another Christmas like this daunted me. I looked back at what I could do then and at what I could do now and I felt far more human and less ill last Christmas, than I do now, just weeks away from Christmas 2013.

When it came to even a simple shopping trip I was out of breath... that was it I decided to stop the Methotrexate... after 3 weeks of the increased dose... much to my GP's disgust. And to be perfectly honest I didn't give a damn what they thought... this was my life and I was beginning to think I knew my own body more than medical science did.

One day we went to Matalan in Strood. By the time I'd got out of the car and walked across the car park, I was breathless. My husband looked at me and said, 'I'm sorry to say this but you are getting worse not better.' I just looked at him and grinned and said, 'Yes my downhill started the day I started to take this Methotrexate.'

That was it, I wasn't taking this anymore, I phoned my consultant's secretary and explained about the breathlessness and the constant relay to the loo and asked if I could increase the Prednisolone if needed until our next visit and stop this Methotrexate. She said she would ask and would get back to me. Luckily for me, his secretary informed by telephone the next day, that it would be OK. I was due back for a consultation on the 11th December 2013, which subsequently got cancelled and rebooked for the 8th January 2014.

Slowly but surely after stopping the Methotrexate I started to have some good days. There isn't a day where I don't ache somewhere or other on my body... but those aches were gradually becoming manageable; in fact I even decreased my own dosage of steroids and I was down to 10mg and 7.5 mg on alternate days.

Yes the fatigue was there still, but not so severe...and whey hey the constant relay trips to and fro the loo was now few and far between. It would only happen now and again (that I could live with)...but according to Google again there is a risk that Prednisolone can cause adverse stomach problems and has been known to cause diarrhea. So perhaps those awful days of spending more time in the loo was an accumulation of side effects of the Methotrexate and the Steroids?

With only about 3 weeks to Christmas, again online shopping was a godsend. Presents ordered and over the course of a few days I wrote the cards... I knew my hands wouldn't manage holding onto a pen and applying pressure to write for long periods of time... but where there is a will there is a way... and doing a few cards a day was the way to go.

Psychologically though, there was a big change in me... it panicked me now to go out alone. I have always been a very independent person... never relied on anyone and never expected other people to care for me, but now I was needy and that frightened the life out of me. I was feeling a burden and no matter how much I was told I wasn't, I still couldn't shake this guilt off. But lately I didn't care... when I went to bed it was just turn the lights out and go...

I am crazy in one way... or so he says, because he has never known anyone to tidy up before going to bed. Yet I have always plumped the cushions put the remote backs on the unit... made sure the sides are tidy in the kitchen... and everything is back in its place. My illogical reasoning was if ever I was burgled in the night, there was no way I was taking the chance of some skanky, low-life, jobless burglar standing in the dock saying my house was a shite-hole when he robbed it.

I can tell you, me being so obstinate at times when I have been ill and doing things, my way, has caused many a row in our house, especially when I have been creased up with a bad back and still got up to do something instead of resting it.

But lately nothing seemed to matter... I didn't care if the housework got done or whether Christmas arrived or not. Even when I had my good days, my interest in things waned. I can't actually say I felt sorry for myself... but I think I had finally reached breaking point and my mind just shut off. Yes if I bumped into people I knew, the false smile would appear and the chat would flow...but deep inside my mind was saying ... how much longer have I got to put up this pretence? Apart from being physically drained... I felt emotionally drained.

'Time to pull yourself together', as my mum would say were the words that were echoing throughout my mind and I brought a Christmas together where the whole family came to me.

Since my mum had her mini-strokes and became house-bound we would visit her Christmas morning and spend time with her but then we would do our own thing... Knowing she was alone at Christmas was something I never really liked deep down. However this year I begged and prayed for her to visit me. I think her seeing the state I was in sometimes when I visited her… gave her the inspiration to try and at least to come me for Christmas Day.

Him indoors, God bless him, knew I was just about coping and cooked the dinner for all us again this year. Yep I pottered about and helped and did the dishing up… but he was the main chef. Mind you though, I think the guests were quite pleased about that, it meant they didn't have to endure my burnt, cremated roast parsnips another year.

Our new edition to the family, with it being his second Christmas, really enjoyed opening his presents and in true kid fashion, left the gifts and played with the boxes. And it bought memories back of when my son was little. And this Christmas we thoroughly enjoyed ourselves… but my body was pleased to see them all go home? You know I don't think they had driven out of the road before I laid my aching body on that sofa and relaxed. As I started to drift off to sleep I only hoped that nobody would knock at the door or ring us on the phone as I don't want to move… not now. Not now I've found comfort at long last.

Boxing day, normally we just laze around and relax… but I wanted to do something different…so I definitely made sure that Christmas day had a whole lot of relaxation in it. My desire was to go to Winter Wonderland in London for Boxing Day. Hubby drove us to Canada Waters where we parked and took a mooch to the Canada Waters Tube Station for the Jubilee line to another tube station and then change tubes so that we arrived at Hyde Park Corner.

The journey up there wasn't bad, but it really showed me how slow I walked. Our son and his girlfriend along with my little soldier in his pushchair, walked at their normal pace… me I was lagging behind already out of breath and thinking to myself this is not a good idea and how stupid I was to even think I would manage a trip to London.

But with a bit of reassurance from my husband and I think he may have even had a word in my son's ear about slowing the pace of the walk down… I managed it. Yes there were not very many places to sit… but there were cafes and bars that had a few seats and a Nordic bar that had plenty of benches to park your ass down on. So I was OK for rest as and when needed.

But I was tiring, my husband could see it… my legs, started their jelly leg feeling and the prospect of having to go through those tubes back to Canada Waters was something I can assure you, I didn't relish. But all in all we had a lovely day, and it just made Christmas that extra bit special. Yes it was a struggle and yes I did pay for it, for a couple of days afterwards, but I would do it all over again.

But then a miracle… I think our little soldier was getting tired and his Nan was definitely flagging, so much so that my husband said…right we will get a black cab to Waterloo and then it is a just a couple of stops on the Jubilee line to Canada Waters and both stations have lifts. Lovely a lift… no struggling on the escalators and all there was to tackle was the short walk to the car.

This is another thing with PMR your legs feel like jelly at times and you feel as if you are going to topple over. A lot of PMR suffers refer to having jelly-leg days. First of all I didn't know what they meant…but I do now.

Standing in pubs all night long or on the banks of the Thames to see in the New Year, is something my mind would love to do but my body knows for full well wouldn't make it, so for us it is New Years Eve, indoors with the TV and Gary Barlow taking us into 2014.

Happy 2014…. Things can only get better.

CHAPTER 11 – THE RINGING IN OF THE NEW YEAR

Here we are lifting our glasses to 2014. Christmas was good and by luck I had a few good days around the Christmas period. I had lowered the dosage of the steroids… something my mind was telling me to do.

I had used Google like everyone else does, to find out all they can about something, normally Google searches are for pleasurable things. However, my searches were more about this illness and finding everything out I could about it and how to cure it, than anything else.

Taking the decorations down was something I didn't relish the thought of. My husband loves his interactive, all singing and dancing festive toys, that are placed all over the lounge and diner. In years to come, I really think we will have to move to get them all in and all working… space is running out at a very rapid rate in this house.

To be perfectly honest at Christmas our home turns into a children's toy shop. Novelty toys on every surface that has a spare space, a 5ft Karaoke Santa and a 6ft Christmas tree and not forgetting the window decorations, so taking decorations down is a mammoth task in itself. Have to say though taking them down is a lot quicker than putting the bloody lot up.

Thank God, he is home until the Monday after New Year, the extra days and his help clearing up after Christmas will be a godsend.

Decorations down, husband back at work, and things seem to be getting back to normal... In fact if anything I haven't felt too bad the last few days...

It was only a few days into January, the 8th to be precise, that my next visit at the hospital was due.

My previous visit apart from being handed more of that Methotrexate wasn't too bad as my consultant was running slightly early. As I walked the corridors of the hospital to the Rheumatology Department I wondered if it would be like the previous visit and I would be seen earlier or whether the waiting room would be packed full of patients like it was when the hospital decided to double book appointments.

As I walked up the corridor towards the booking in desk, I saw on my consultant's door the words, *'Running on Time'* brilliant I thought I can be out of here quite quick then.

I don't think I had managed to park my ass before my name was called. I thought it might have been to fill in one of these forms again, but no it was to see the consultant.

He is a nice man, but… oh yes there always has to be a big but about something…doesn't there? To me he doesn't seem to explain things that thoroughly and you feel rather rushed at times. Anyway he asked how I was feeling and I said I was having my good days and my bad days and I still ached but slowly since Christmas those aches have been less severe… and that I had managed to get myself down to 7.5mg of Prednisolone, which he was pleased about, but I told him the aches were returning a little today.

He told me that he wanted me off of Prednisolone and he gave me a reduction chart on how to lower the dosage. And it must be done by taking different doses on alternative days until I am on 5mg daily.

Then came the shock of the appointment, oh yes there always has to be one. And mine was the consultant telling me there is another bloody drug that they use to treat this disease and that he wants me to start taking it. This time I have to take 10mg daily and after two weeks increase it to 20mg until my next visit in 6 months. Armed once again, with three, butchering blood test forms, a prescription for 1mg Prednisolone and now this new drug called Leflunomide, a drug that is used to reduce the inflammation caused by some auto-immune diseases, I left the hospital thinking here we go again.

Mind you I didn't make the same mistake as I did before…I did remember to stop off at the Out-Patients Booking-in desk and make my next appointment. Perhaps I am not going senile after all?

To save me dragging myself out to the chemist, normally I ring through, order my medication and then hubby picks it up on his way home from work. But now there was another tablet to be ordered, so the prescription needed to be dropped into the chemist. I was told, by him of higher descent…or so he likes to believe… that I was to get a cab up that morning to the hospital and one back. Normally the thought of spending a fortune on taxis whilst the bus is at the bottom of the hill, makes me go into Scrooge mode. No way am I going to pay that price when I can get a bus and change at Chatham. Plus the fact it is nice to talk to people, at the bus stop, that is after inspecting them at close quarters to see if they have Chicken Pox or Shingles or whether they could be harbouring the next generation of the plague.

So decision made, I need to take this prescription to the chemist, so it is a bus to Chatham, then change off that bus to one that takes me to the bottom of the road where the chemist is and one to bring me back up the hill.

Yes along my road, and down the hill and you reach the chemist. Not far just a few minutes' walk…or a lot of minutes for me going at snail's pace. But it is a form of exercise even if it is just the walk down there. But as of late the thought of having to climb the hill sends my body into anaphylactic shock. The agony it is to climb hills is no nobody's business so the option that was left to me was after I went into the chemist I would then get the bus up the hill.

Finally, I staggered into the chemist and handed in the prescription... the girl behind the counter, says, 'You are definitely going to rattle soon, if you haven't already.'

Then the problems started, there was something not right with the prescription, however I think the Pharmacist realised that if he didn't sort it out... this customer could go into meltdown or drop down dead at the thought of having to go back to the hospital to sort it out... Anyway they took the prescription and sorted the problem and then told me that they wouldn't be able to get the medication in until the afternoon of the next day.

I had another prescription ordered that was due back at the chemist on the Friday so I told the Pharmacist that it would be perfectly OK and I will collect both prescriptions either Friday night or Saturday morning.

Now for the trip home… do I or don't I? I took one look at the hill that leads up to my road and remembered back to the last time I thought I had the stamina and capability of walking up that hill. How embarrassing it was… I got overtook by a woman with a walking stick and dragging a shopping trolley…who was a good few years older than me. The sheer embarrassment of this for that moment had me leaning on someone's wall and having hysterics… oh pray I do hope, I can stop laughing soon and I hope I don't pee myself… but there she was with her stick and trolley climbing this hill with no problems… and there I was struggling like I was just about to die of exhaustion. Steroids they say give you energy… well could somebody tell the ones I am taking what they are supposed to do that…because if anything I am very short of bloody energy or more to the point have no bloody energy whatsoever. There I was trying to stem my laughter, when I looked over the road and there was a workman with his barrow, moving stuff in one of the gardens. For a minute I bet he wondered what was wrong with me, but to be honest, I think if he had at that precise moment come across and asked what was wrong, I would have promptly asked him for a lift up the hill on his barrow.

So the decision was made, the prospect of me making that hill was a definite no-no... so back down the road, to the bus stop and catch the bus.

Home, safe and sound, without wetting myself, thank God, and still chuckling away as I reminisced about day I saw that OAP who must have been on speed, climb that hill. She must have been. I have never seen anyone climb that hill that fast. Doc... give me what she is having... please.

After my troop around, I didn't feel too bad and thought I will wake up aching tomorrow.

Correct.

I woke up, not just aching but without a friggin voice. The dogs thought I was playing a silly game as I squeaked at them. People phoned and then hung up and rang back... my mother who has terrible trouble hearing on the telephone, was now practically frantic thinking she had an heavy-breathing nutter, talking dirty to her, shouting, 'Is that you Bren?' With me trying to get out the word... YES to no avail. After she stuffed her hearing aid further into her ear she managed to realise it was me and she was not the victim of some dirty pervert trying to get his jollies.

As Thursday progressed, the cold started to come out... surely this couldn't be the Christmas cold my son had developed... not after all this time. Or did someone on that bus have a bug? I knew I should have said as I got on the buses... 'Will all infected passengers please ascend to the upper deck.' Mind you that would have been funny because one of those vehicles I travelled on that day was a coach...poor sods would have had to sit on the roof in the pouring rain. Well at least I might have still had a voice.

Friday ... still no voice. And neither did I have a sore throat... just a runny nose and no voice.

Saturday morning came and still no voice. Finally my mum could talk to someone who she could hear when they spoke. Hubby went to the chemist for me, and collected the barrow-load of drugs. One for blood pressure, one antihistamine, the steroids, the anti-inflammatory, and the new drug, the Amitriptyline for my back and of course the painkillers.

Luckily this new drug you don't have to take with food, unlike the steroids… which now I take now after a couple of hours after I have woken up and instead of heaving at a bowl of Frosties, I found it much easier to munch 3 Go-Ahead biscuits. Plus the fact that I think they are very tasty.

So here we are on the 11th January 2014 and the start of the new tablets. The apprehension and fear is there at the back of my mind even though I don't have a voice… you see, since stopping the Methotrexate I am not having a full-time affair with our loo now and I don't want to be back to the stage of spending more time with Andrex than other people.

Well pills down neck and now it is just a matter of time to see if they agree with me or not. Voice or no voice… I wanted to get out of this house…I might have no voice, but I don't feel too bad… so we decided to pop out for a couple of hours. Then upon returning home… a letter on the door mat from my GP… asking me to contact the surgery and get an appointment.

Now that was hilarious, trying to phone up on Monday morning to get an appointment with no voice. Through the squeaks, the receptionist managed to book me an appointment in for Thursday afternoon. She told me it was nothing to worry about, just a medical review and to see how I got on at the hospital.

Tuesday came and words started to sound like proper words and not some mish mash of squeaks…and I wasn't feeling too bad… I took a look around and thought my God this house does need a good old clean… so topped myself up with painkillers and set about it. I must have overdone it, because that night my muscles in my right leg were playing havoc and I had a sharp pain in my hip. When the other half came in and saw me hobbling about again, did I get told off? I felt like a really naughty child. But deep down there was some self-satisfaction that I had managed to clean the house.

Wednesday, the voice was back in full flow... but the hip was nowhere near getting better... it hurt to turn my leg... and the pain and burning sensation was right down the back of my leg... bollox ... sciatica now deciding to put in an appearance.

Thursday I was due at the Doctors, honestly over the last few days I am sure if I had been a horse I would have been shot. It would have been the humane thing to do.

I walked in, and it was the review of the blood pressure... yep you guessed it, it was high. We spoke about the new drug the hospital gave me and he again told me, just like the hospital I will need to be monitored, and have regular blood tests due to the fact that this drug can affect your liver and kidneys.

After a few minutes he tried the blood pressure again, to see if it had lowered at all, but no it was just the same. One of the things that this new drug can do, is elevate your blood pressure. The Doctor didn't want to risk it going any higher as by the weekend after next I was to increase the dosage. So that was it.. another bloody drug prescribed... this time a water tablet that helps to combat blood pressure.

To think how much this would cost me, if I had to pay the full prescription amount of £7.85 per item, would set me back at least £78.50 a month as some of the drugs I take have to be in different strengths. Thankfully though I registered for the Yearly Prepayment Card at £104 a year, which you can pay via a monthly direct debit. Being ill is costly... I wonder how some people manage to pay for prescriptions especially if two or three items are prescribed... without the Pre-Payment scheme I know for a fact I couldn't afford to find nearly £80 a month.

Now January has another week to go before we are into February and already I can feel my immune system taking a bashing. The no energy feeling is back, but that could be because my hip is still giving me jip at times... but I don't feel as good as I did before...

Now which tablet is not agreeing with me? Is it the Leflunomide or is it the water tablet... I have noticed that if I get up suddenly I feel giddy and woozy for a minute... but could that be where my blood pressure is a little low.. Think I will give it to the end of the following month and then decide whether or not to stop taking this Leflunomide... because I don't think a water tablet would cause too many problems.

In fact I think if things don't change by the end of February, I am going to wean myself off of the steroids and take my bloody chances... I think I felt better before I went to the hospital initially. I know my immune system is taking a battering because I have never had so many festers on my fingers... as soon as I catch the side of my finger near the nail and the skin breaks... and I am a nail biter, always have and always will be – within a matter of days a fester will appear. Since Christmas I have had to burst three of them... 7 more to go and then I can say I've had a handful. Who knows what the future holds... but things can only get better can't they?

CHAPTER 12 – SUNDAY 26TH JANUARY 2014

Today is the day that I have decided to conclude entries for this book. On Saturday 11th January 2014; I started the first dose of 10mg of the new tablet, Leflunomide, issued by the hospital. For 14 days I took religiously 10mg and last night was the start of the 20mg dose. I know I have been ill with a cold and loss of voice and my hip has been playing up but I don't feel well again.

I feel lethargic and my concentration levels just about peak above zero. Times are slipping through my mind… you know only this afternoon I was on my way upstairs to get the next lot of washing, stopped off to have a pee, and then promptly slumped back onto the sofa… minus the washing.

WTF?

How can you forget what you are supposed to be doing, by just having a pee break? This is not normal, that is for sure.

Concentration levels zero, jelly legs definitely.

To be honest I thought this new drug might have no side-effects but no I am beginning to have recollections of how that Methotrexate made me feel initially… Please not this time…not with this drug.

Yesterday was the start of the increased dosage…I wasn't feeling too good and thought perhaps because I was taking the medication in the morning the side effects were because of the drug being taken on an empty stomach, even though the instruction leaflet said you can take it with or without food. It certainly isn't agreeing with me without food that is for sure. So my plan of action was, take it after our evening meal and then perhaps all those side effects would occur whilst I was sleeping.

No friggin way was that going to happen.

1am came and 1am passed, sleepy no… tired yes. 2am came and went just like 1am; finally at gone 3am in the morning I knew I would be able to sleep.

Finally I fell to sleep…and rose at 10.45am today, shattered, lethargic and with the most horrendous mouth… You know the one, the one where you have the hangover of all hangovers and your mouth feels like a gorilla's armpit.

I wouldn't have minded so much, if I had been having a night on the tiles. But through medication! This is getting bloody stupid and I am fed up to the back teeth of it.

Of course, today, hasn't got any better, I still feel like I did yesterday and now I have altered the time of the new dosage it seems I will have to continue until I manage to miss one day and go back to taking it in the morning.

Drugs and me have always had a row…I am allergic to Penicillin, and anti-inflammatory drugs, cause me a severe attack of irritable bowel.

Naturally when you are not feeling on top of the world, something has to happen just to add to your stress levels. Well our son decided today to come home from his girlfriend's home earlier than usual… Hubby again was lumbered with cooking the dinner and was just in the process of dishing it up, when our son bought in our little soldier to say hello…of course the dogs went ballistic as per usual. When you have light carpets and 8 paws to mop up, when the weather turns foul you resort to shutting the baby gate.

From the moment the dogs arrived, we decided to put a baby gate between the kitchen and lounge, which gets shut at night at bedtime. Of course the weather today has done nothing but rain, so the mop bucket has been out time and time again, and at this moment was standing by the cupboard and the safety gate.

Yep, you guessed it, the doggies were hanging over the baby gate wanting to lick little man to death as he was being held in father's arms, when our Dumpling decided to put her rear foot in the mop bucket and send it scuttling over the kitchen… water everywhere.

That was it…dinner was put on hold… and one mass mop-up started. I tried my hardest to help, but I was more of a hindrance than help. Eventually we got most of the water up and he used the mop and I got the Hoover Wet and Dry hand-held cleaner out… but that was running on very low batteries so it was struggling sucking up the water. Then the tears welled up in my eyes…all because I wanted to remove the canister holding the water as it was nearly full and couldn't. No matter how hard I tried no way could I get the bloody thing that holds the water off the hoover… gradually the water was spilling out all over the place… frustration came over me…I could have thrown the bloody thing. But he came and sorted it out. Then when I emptied I didn't have the strength to put it back together… Oh FFS. Here I was now throwing more water around the bloody kitchen than the dogs did in the first place. No wonder he looks at me at times in despair.

I could well imagine the conversation my hands were having between themselves.

'Do you really think you are going to have the strength to get that off lady? No bitch, leftie and I have decided to let you down… we do like to see your suffer as you struggle.'

We dried the floor up as best as we could and left the back door open to dry the floor whilst we had our dinner. Then the loading of the dishwasher… I could multitask, like most women do without batting an eye, with no problems beforehand. Not now. Multitasking and I are now a thing of the past...like an ex...good at the time but a right swine since you dumped them.

The only two things that needed doing, was to put the washing in the dryer and load the dishwasher... Not rocket science, is it? Simple tasks, really but not when you don't feel well and feel confused and can't think straight.

Eventually I just stood at the dishwasher with the washing machine door open ready to move the stuff and for that moment I couldn't think straight... thank God for superhero hubby, who said, 'Bugger off in there and I'll do it.'

Now as the evening approaches I am starting to feel a little more human.

I know it can't be my blood pressure tablet causing this because I've been taking it for years with no problems... The anti-inflammatory never made me feel as if I was nothing but a zombie. Could the real problem be the steroids? Oh my how do I get off of these bloody things? I know you just can't stop taking them, because of the effect they have on your adrenal glands. So what is the best way to do it? I think the only option is to lower them as the hospital says, but instead of keeping on the 5mg until my next visit in July, I will copy his plan and lower the dosage until I am off of them.

Unless PMR does make you feel like this…my plan of action might not be the correct one. But it is one that I am now going to try. Those few days at Christmas when I felt great were wonderful… I just want those days back again. And here we go again, I feel tired, but can't sleep. Another late night I suspect.

CHAPTER 13 – GUILT AND THE LOW ESTEEM

It is really hard to put into words how this disease affects you, not just physically but mentally. Put it this way... when you have a sore throat you know within a couple of days it will be less sore and by the end of the week, you will more than likely be fine.

Just like if you slip and break an ankle... there is a very good chance that after 6 weeks in plaster and a few weeks of physiotherapy you will be good enough to do the light fantastic.

Even flu has a time limitation on it, unless of course you suffer further complications, like a chest infection... but PMR? No there is no time limit to how long it lasts and it plagues some people for years. The doctors always say that within a couple of years you will be back fighting fit just like your old self... but that isn't true. There are people on the likes of Facebook, in groups, that have suffered a whole lot longer than two years... some even coming close to double figures with regards to the number of years they have been suffering with this dreaded disease.

It is not one of these things, where you think, 'I feel like fucking shite, but I know will be OK to go to Gloria's Tupperware party next week.'

You don't know how you are going to feel from one day to the next. You might have quite a few days, where you feel as bright as a button and then wham bam, you are back to feeling like you have just been pulled through a wringer and pushed back through it.

People look at you and they can see you sniff, and they can hear your voice has gone. They can't see spots and they can't see anything physically wrong with you, so they assume that what you are suffering from is just a few aches and pains… which every person gets, especially as they get older. What they don't realise is that it is not the normal aches and pains that subside with rest and a couple of paracetamol… it is muscular pain and inflammation, that has decided it is moving into your cosy body and there is no way it is leaving you because to leave you means that it has to take up residence in sub-standard accommodation that is not fit for rats to live in yet alone humans.

And even if we are not in pain, we have to deal with the bloody side-effects that come with the drugs we take that stop us being in pain. We might not look sick on the outside but inside we are... Sometimes the battle is not just about dealing with the disease but it is the uphill battle of dealing with all the drugs we take and their friggin side effects.

When people ask how you are... 'Fine' is what we say, because you see we don't look ill, and if we did tell you how we really felt... deep down we know that it would be so hard for a person to believe, how someone looking not so bad on the outside can be so ill on the inside.... PMR is the invisible illness.

I found this picture on Facebook and I think all those words listed, I have felt at one time or another.

"How are you?"

Broken. Useless. Alone. Clueless. Confused. Betrayed. Fragile. On the verge of tears. Depressed. Anxious. About to break down. Really given up. Pathetic. Annoying. I'm just a burden. Distant. Lonely. Bitter. Heartbroken. Lovely. Rejected. Crushed. I feel like I'm going to just fall apart at any moment. Empty. Defeated. Never good enough.

Fine.

Useless - Oh yes I have felt that… especially when I can't stretch to reach things, or I can't open a bottle that has been previously opened but someone has tightened the lid just that little too tight for my weak fingers.

When you try to do the simplest of tasks, it can be a chore, people around you tend to try to hold onto their patience but you can see it is in their eyes, you can see their thoughts, 'Oh FFS give it here, we'll be all night waiting for you to do it.' As much as their mouths don't say the words that you know they must be thinking, their facial expressions do.

You can't blame them because deep down you know you'd feel the same but my God it does knock you back.

I'm just a burden – Oh yes most definitely one of the most poignant feelings ever. When you have to ask people to do this that and the other… things that you used to do and do so easily. Carrying the hoover upstairs for instance… or can you just whip the hoover around the floor and pick the dog's hairs up. Then that brings in the feeling of being useless and no matter how many times your loves ones tell you that you are not a burden you know you are…You are fed up with yourself so it is only natural that others will be too. You have hell of a lot time to think, and think to yourself, they must be fed up with me… what can I do to ease this burden on them?

Those awful thoughts enter your head, and you think about whether those close to you would they would have a better quality of life if you were not there with them. Your mind goes into the depths of are they just there, with you, because people wouldn't think highly of them if they upped sticks and left.

This is your illness and not theirs, and I know you make those vows of in sickness as in health…but there is a limit to what any person should have to endure.

Guilty – one that isn't listed above in that picture that really does need to be there… when you suffer from a disease that leaves you in chronic pain, it isn't just you it affects. It affects everyone around you, you husband, your kids and your friends. You carry this guilt within you that it must be your fault that you are like this. You must have done something so wrong somewhere and this is your comeuppance. You seriously must have pissed him up there off real big time.

But the feeling of guilt that your family now have to suffer is the worst to live with. They married you… they didn't marry PMR and they don't deserve this. I am one of the lucky ones, my husband understands and he cares, but I know it takes its toll on him sometimes. His patience gets a bit frayed especially if I am doing something, and I am fumbling away… that is when he will but in… take over and do it so easily… and that is when the guilt feeling hits home. That is when the tears want to flow.. that is when I want to scream out aloud, but instead I just take those feelings and hide them deep down inside me and say nowt. I know he doesn't mean to be so abrasive but it does make me feel so guilty... it makes me think this is my fault... and at times bloody sorry for myself.

Depressed – Yep been there, done that and got the T-Shirt as they say. Depression sets in so easily... even though I suffered for years with a bad back and sciatica, with attacks that would send me to my bed for a couple of days, none of those pains prepared me for how much agony PMR was going to bring me... Large muscle weakness, large muscle pain, shoulders aching, neck feeling as if it was just about to snap. Not being mobile, and seeing people older than you, have a better quality of life inevitably makes you depressed. You try your hardest to shake it... but when one day just merges into another with no change... depression takes its hold.

One thing I have to say, in my fight against it, I was born with a very strong character which I have kept throughout my life and I will not succumb to depression. When I know it is getting too much… I give myself a good firm talking too, shed those tears and have my private 'I feel sorry for myself' moment and boldly refuse to go any further into the depths of despair.

Bitter – most definitely at times. Why me? What have I done so wrong? But bitterness can lead to depression so again I give myself a swift kick up the backside and bring myself together. Mind you having two Golden Retrievers give you a lick and their unconditional love soon makes those deepest darkest moments, tolerable to bear. But I can understand how people feel and how they feel as if they've been short-changed and have drawn the short straw of life.

Anxious – Anxious, apprehensive, scared to death and fear all rolled into one descends upon you like very heavy smog with zero visibility. You can't see an end to the illness and days that incapacitate you to the point of where all you do is think about the future… and how bleak it looks. The fear of what could happen and how you will cope when you are older sends shockwaves of anxiousness through your body. The thought of ending up in a wheelchair or just lying in a bed is something that you dread the most. You can't help but get anxious at times. And those around you just don't seem to understand how you feel deep inside. You try to explain, but the words can't find their way out of your mouth, so you suffer in silence. You don't want to worry people and you don't want sympathy but you fear by telling others of your deepest darkest thoughts will either make them think you a either a fruit-bat or plain right bloody pathetic.

Defeated – Yes there are times when you feel totally defeated, you are battered and bruised both physically and mentally… You feel as if you are fighting a constant war against what you body is doing and you are losing every battle. Then to keep you going, you win a battle or two and then the nightmare starts all over again.

You get to that point where you want to throw the towel in, scream and shout and say… 'Fuck you PMR, you win.' But you can't. There is no safe place where you and your body can escape to, so that this disease leaves you alone for a while. You long for the day, when you get up feeling like a young gazelle and able to do what you want to do, without fear of pain putting the dampner on what you are enjoying so much. And when that day doesn't arrive you just feel like throwing in the towel. You are deflated, defeated and totally depressed.

Low self-esteem – believe me that one is hard to deal with... When your immune system is shot away, apart from having to deal with your swollen Prednisolone face, you have to deal with hair that looks limp, lank, dull, and would need a vat of ready-mix concrete to give those roots a slim chance of having some volume. All the products on the shelf don't put that sheen back into your hair... I think at times you would get better results with a spray of Pledge polish than an expensive can of spray that is supposed to add gloss to your hair and give it the ultimate shine that you have been longing for.

It isn't the product that is failing or duff... because you know you have used it before and it worked great...it is the immune system sapping all the goodness out of everything it can, your hair, your skin, your nail, your complexion, every bloody thing gets affected.

When you look in the mirror and see yourself staring back and know that your weight has ballooned because of Prednisolone because it increases your appetite and if you starve yourself you feel even worse, that is when the downer really hits you. People around you don't say anything, but you can see their glares, they must think my God, she has let herself go, believe me I haven't. It is just a case of the medication, the illness, has these horrible effects on my external appearance… Yes my hair doesn't look like it did before the illness, but it is hardly my bloody fault is it?

Don't judge me please or any other sufferer of PMR for that matter, just walk in our shoes for a while and then see how you feel. Strap a tin of beans to your arms and then do your daily chores… it won't be long before that tin of beans feels like you have strapped a crate of beans to your arms. And your arms feel like lead, ache like hell and have no strength to them. The only difference is you can remove that can of beans when you want… we can't.

When you hands and fingers ache, try putting pegs on your fingers and carrying on with your chores and see how much and how long you can do your normal chores. That is how our hands ache, especially if you're suffering PMR and wear and tear of the joints, as well as suffering from the likes of osteoarthritis.

And no I am not feeling sorry for myself… but anyone that doesn't understand a disease like PMR or Fibromyalgia or any other immune disease, that affects your body inwardly… really should learn that we didn't ask for this… we had no choice, and if today it was a choice of giving up a lottery win and having your health back or taking the money and living with PMR, I, for one, would gladly hand the cash back… and so would you if you had to deal with this shite day in and day out whilst not knowing how long for. But one thing I do know is this, sometimes you have some very deep and dark moments. Moments were your mind goes to places where you would never ever dream of going.

I have always said that if I was senile padded up like a baby and not knowing who the hell was who... I would opt for a dignified death. I have said that if I got cancer I wouldn't want my family to see me in agony and laying there just waiting for that next morphine injection that was now so strong in order to deal with the pain that it killed me.

But the prospect of having to live with this for the rest of my life... frightens me to death. The fear that it won't get any better and it will only get worse, scares me to death. The thought of getting to the stage where my only mode of transport is a wheelchair is something I don't want to ever happen. Those thoughts scare me and even though my body is acting like it is on its last legs... my mind is still as young as it was when I was 18. A little bit wiser but still as mentally active as I was all those years ago, when I was able to dance the night away, with high-heels still attached to feet... sleep for 4 hours and then do a full day's work, before I came home and did it all that partying all over again.

I yearn for those days to return, but then realise that is not going to happen. PMR affects a lot of people and people who live with chronic pain day in and day out do have a cross to bear.

Making plans is something that we so want to do but know that when we are in the full midst of a flare-up of the symptoms, the most we are going to do that day or until the symptoms subside is just the bare necessities.

You think you are coming to terms with the side-effects of the drugs and then another reaction occurs or the drugs you are taking don't agree with you or they are not making you any better, so you are back to square one of trying a new medication and having to deal with the side-effects all over again, not knowing if you are firstly going to get any and if you do are they going to be as severe as the side effects you had on the other drug.

What the future holds for me, I don't know… whether I could be writing a sequel next year, telling people how I am still coping with this debilitating disease or whether I might be one of

those lucky ones and go into a remission that has no flare-ups, I don't know.
I suppose only time will tell…..

RESOURCES

Polymyalgia Rheumatica – Arthritis Research UK

Polymyalgia Rheumatica (usually shortened to PMR) is an inflammatory condition that causes many (poly) painful muscles (myalgia), mainly in your shoulder and thigh.

PMR can start at any age from 50 but mainly affects people over the age of 60. Women are affected 2–3 times as often as men and it affects about 1 in 2,000

Download of booklet

Giant Cell Arteritis – Arthritis Research UK

Giant cell arteritis (usually shortened to GCA) is one of a group of conditions referred to as vasculitis, meaning inflammation in the blood vessels.

It's called an arteritis because it affects the arteries rather than the veins. It commonly affects the arteries of the skull, causing pain and tenderness over the temples. Because of this, GCA is often known as temporal arteritis

<u>Download of booklet</u>

<u>Polymyalgia Rheumatica – American College of Rheumatology</u> (PDF)

Polymyalgia Rheumatica (sometimes referred to as PMR) is a common cause of wide spread aching and stiffness in older adults. Because PMR does not often cause swollen joints, it may be hard to recognize.

PMR may occur with another health problem, Giant Cell Arteritis.

<u>What are Steroids – Arthritis Research UK</u>

Some steroids occur naturally in your body. Man-made steroids act like natural steroids to reduce inflammation. They can be given in tablet form or as an injection. A steroid mixture can be injected into and around an inflamed joint to ease your symptoms. It's called a local injection because it acts in a particular area.

[Download the booklet on steroid tablets](#)

[Download the booklet on steroid local injections](#)

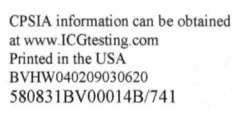